# BRADY

# EMT REVIEW: EXAMINATION PREPARATION

*Third Edition*

## Thomas C. Hanes
## Carolyn C. Hanes

Brady
*A Prentice Hall Division*
Englewood Cliffs, New Jersey 07632

**Library of Congress Cataloging-in-Publication Data**

Hanes, Carolyn C.
    EMT review : examination preparation / Carolyn C. Hanes, Thomas C. Hanes.—3rd ed.
      p. cm.
    "A Brady book."
    ISBN 0-89303-730-3
    1. Medical emergencies—Examinations, questions, etc. I. Hanes, Thomas C. II. Title.
    [DNLM: 1. Allied Health Personnel—examination questions. 2. Emergencies—examination questions. 3. Emergency Medical Services—examination questions. 4. First Aid—examination questions. WX 18 H237e]
RC86.9.H36 1991
616.02'5'076—dc20
DNLM/DLC
for Library of Congress
                                    90-14256
                                           CIP

Editorial/production supervision and
   interior design: Tally Morgan, WordCrafters
Cover design: Ben Santora
Prepress buyer: Mary McCartney
Manufacturing buyer: Ed O'Dougherty
Acquisitions editor: Natalie Anderson

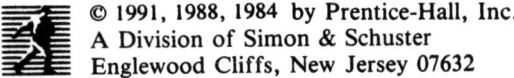
© 1991, 1988, 1984 by Prentice-Hall, Inc.
A Division of Simon & Schuster
Englewood Cliffs, New Jersey 07632

All rights reserved. No part of this book may be
reproduced, in any form or by any means,
without permission in writing from the publisher.

Printed in the United States of America
10 9 8 7 6 5 4 3

ISBN 0-89303-730-3

Prentice-Hall International (UK) Limited, *London*
Prentice-Hall of Australia Pty. Limited, *Sydney*
Prentice-Hall Canada Inc., *Toronto*
Prentice-Hall Hispanoamericana, S.A., *Mexico*
Prentice-Hall of India Private Limited, *New Delhi*
Prentice-Hall of Japan, Inc., *Tokyo*
Simon & Schuster Asia Pts. Ltd., *Singapore*
Editora Prentice-Hall do Brasil, Ltda., *Rio de Janeiro*

# Contents

| | | | |
|---|---|---|---|
| | Introduction, **v** | **Unit 18-I** | Environmental Emergencies |
| **Unit 1** | The Emergency Medical Technician, **1** | | Section One: Heat- and Cold-Related Emergencies, **113** |
| **Unit 2** | The Human Body, **5** | **Unit 18-II** | Environmental Emergencies |
| **Unit 3** | Patient Assessment, **10** | | Section Two: Water- and Ice-Related Accidents, **116** |
| **Unit 4** | Basic Life Support I: The Airway and Pulmonary Resuscitation, **15** | **Unit 19** | Special Patients and Behavioral Problems, **119** |
| **Unit 5** | Basic Life Support II: CPR—Cardiopulmonary Resuscitation, **20** | **Unit 20** | Triage and Disaster Management, **123** |
| **Unit 6** | Breathing Aids and Oxygen Therapy, **31** | **Unit 21** | Preparing for the Ambulance Run, **128** |
| **Unit 7-I** | Basic Life Support III: Bleeding and Shock | **Unit 22** | Responding to the Call for Help, **129** |
| | *Section 1: Basic Procedures*, **38** | **Unit 23** | Transferring Patients to the Ambulance, **132** |
| **Unit 7-II** | Basic Life Support III | **Unit 24** | Transporting the Patient to a Hospital, **138** |
| | *Section 2: Pneumatic Counterpressure Devices—The Anti-Shock Garment*, **45** | **Unit 25** | Terminating the Run, **143** |
| **Unit 8** | Injuries I: Soft Tissues and Internal Organs, **49** | **Unit 26** | Communications and Reports, **144** |
| **Unit 9** | Injuries II: Musculoskeletal Injuries—The Upper Extremities, **56** | **Unit 27-I** | Vehicle Rescue Section One: Equipment for Vehicle Rescue, **145** |
| **Unit 10** | Injuries II: The Lower Extremities, **60** | **Unit 27-II** | Vehicle Rescue Section Two: Managing Accident-Related Hazards, **146** |
| **Unit 11** | Injuries III: The Skull and Spine, **63** | | |
| **Unit 12** | Injuries III: Soft Tissue Injuries of the Head and Neck, **67** | **Unit 27-III** | Vehicle Rescue Section Three: Gaining Access to Vehicle Occupants, **148** |
| **Unit 13** | Injuries IV: The Chest, Abdomen, and Genitalia, **76** | | |
| **Unit 14-I** | Medical Emergencies—Section 1, **81** | **Unit 27-IV** | Vehicle Rescue Section Four: Disentangling Trapped Persons, **150** |
| **Unit 14-II** | Medical Emergencies—Section 2, **91** | | |
| **Unit 15** | Pediatric Emergencies, **95** | | |
| **Unit 16** | Childbirth, **100** | **Unit 28** | Sample Final Examination, **153** |
| **Unit 17** | Burns and Hazardous Materials, **108** | **Answers, 162** | |

*Dedication*
To Christianne and Jonathan

# Introduction

Becoming an EMT in today's technological age is clearly not an easy task. The days of poorly trained technicians and the "haul and run" methodology have been replaced with the new technology and a better trained emergency medical technician. Today's EMT student must assimilate volumes of information and be able to sort out and put together many signs, symptoms, contraindications, and treatments. For many, classroom and study habits have long since become memories. This text attempts to allow you to make mistakes now, before the patient suffers later in real life.

*EMT Review: Examination Preparation* is designed to be used by the basic-level EMT student as a self-paced review manual, in close harmony with the course textbook. It is not intended to replace in-class quizzes, tests, or practical exams. Although geared to the first-time EMT student, this text may also be used by EMTs preparing for recertification examinations.

Both multiple choice questions and practical situations from each chapter of *Emergency Care, Fifth Edition* are presented. The answer key at the end of each chapter gives the correct answer and a direct page reference to *Emergency Care, Fifth Edition*. The answer key also supplies a reference to two other texts, *Emergency Care and Transportation of the Sick and Injured*, Fourth Edition. The student should be advised that the questions were drawn directly from *Emergency Care*, Fifth Edition, and that conflicts exist between the textbooks. Where appropriate, the answer key will point out the conflicts as well as indicate questions that cannot be answered by the *Emergency Care and Transportation of the Sick and Injured* text.

A sample final examination is provided to help the EMT student prepare for the course final exam as well as the state and national examinations.

We have attempted to provide multiple choice questions that do not contain negative stems in the main body of the question, since the negative stem often is overlooked by the student. "All of the above" and "None of the above" responses also have not been included, since these usually are giveaways to the correct answer.

It is beyond the scope of this text to attempt to teach you how to prepare for and take tests. A few general suggestions are:

1. Read the chapter objectives first.

2. Skim over the chapter quickly, then reread the chapter carefully while taking notes.

3. Take the appropriate test in this book.

4. Read each question carefully, then look for key words or the central point of the question.

5. Do not read extra meaning into the question.

6. Eliminate obvious incorrect answers.

7. If more than one answer looks correct, make a note in the margin of your answer sheet and continue on to the next question.

8. Reread the skipped questions after you have answered all other questions.

9. Do not spend too much time on any one question.

The test format in this text groups questions according to common topic for each unit as well as for the sample final examination. This grouping should allow those students having difficulty to keep their thoughts from jumping around from topic to topic.

The practical exercises at the end of each unit are designed for the student to develop an approach to assess the patient's condition and to develop a method of stabilization, transportation, and continuing care en route to the emergency room. Although designed to be answered by the student and then reviewed by the instructor, these situations may be used to set up practical situations for review in class.

C.C.H.
T.C.H.

# 1

# The Emergency Medical Technician

- *Emergency Medical Services System*
- *The Emergency Medical Technician*
- *The EMT and the Law*
- *Equipment*
- *National Organizations*

---

1. Once the EMT begins care for a person who has had an accident, or for a person who is ill, that person is referred to:

    a. as a victim.
    b. as a patient.
    c. by first name only.
    d. only by last name.

2. One of the biggest mistakes made by new EMTs is:

    a. using neutral conversation.
    b. using inappropriate conversation.
    c. providing care above the level of their training.
    d. remaining calm.

3. The minimum accepted care based on state laws, administrative orders, and locally accepted procedures set up by emergency care organizations is called:

    a. liability.
    b. total patient care.
    c. the good samaritan law.
    d. the standard of care.

4. Saying to a patient who has just wrecked a new car and has broken his leg, "Relax, everything is all right. There's nothing to worry about," is an example of:

    a. the standard of care.
    b. appropriate, calm, neutral conversation.
    c. inappropriate conversation.
    d. total patient care.

5. An EMT can be sued and held liable for:

    a. refusing to treat a patient due to lack of consent.
    b. providing care above the level of the training.
    c. forcing care upon an incompetent adult who has refused care.
    d. treating a severely injured child even though the parents are not present to grant consent.

6. If the parents or legal guardians of a child sustaining life-threatening injuries are not at the scene and can not be reached, the EMT may assume:

    a. informed consent is granted.
    b. actual consent is granted.
    c. implied consent is granted.
    d. consent is refused.

## 2  THE EMERGENCY MEDICAL TECHNICIAN

7. Once you stop to help someone in a medical emergency, you have legally initiated care. If you leave this patient before completing care or handing over care to someone with at least your level of training, you may be subject to legal action due to:

   a. the medical practices act.
   b. the good samaritan act.
   c. abandonment.
   d. implied consent.

8. The emergency medical record, which contains information gathered while assessing and monitoring a patient, is:

   a. a legal document.
   b. a public record.
   c. of little importance.
   d. recorded in the EMT's notebook.

9. Care for mentally disturbed patients usually is provided under the laws of:

   a. refused consent.
   b. implied consent.
   c. informed consent.
   d. actual consent.

10. An ambulance that has a forward cab and an integral body with a walk-through compartment is called a:

    a. type I ambulance.
    b. type II ambulance.
    c. type III ambulance.
    d. type IV ambulance.

11. When the EMT has received oral consent to treat a conscious, mentally competent adult, this is called:

    a. actual consent.
    b. implied consent.
    c. immunity from liability.
    d. total patient care.

12. Informed consent, which indicates that the patient knows who you are, your level of training and certification, what is wrong, and how you plan to treat him or her, is best obtained:

    a. by having the patient sign a consent form.
    b. orally, so as not to waste time.
    c. only for mentally incompetent patients.
    d. only for minors.

13. A child has been bitten by a neighbor's dog. Upon arrival, the EMT should:

    a. kill the animal at once.
    b. check the animal for rabies.
    c. prevent others from being bitten by dog.
    d. find the owner of the dog.

14. If a person is found unconscious or so ill or badly injured that his or her judgement is impaired, the EMT should assume that the victim wishes to be treated. The legal basis for this action is called:

    a. applied consent.
    b. refused consent.
    c. conditional consent.
    d. implied consent.

15. If you are at the scene of an accident but leave to answer another call before other help arrives:

    a. you cannot be held liable.
    b. this is abandonment and you may be held liable.
    c. this is abandonment only if life-threatening emergencies exist.
    d. this is abandonment if the second call involves less serious injuries.

16. During transportation of an emotionally disturbed female, the patient should:

    a. be treated no differently than any male patient.
    b. never be physically restrained.
    c. never be transported without police approval.
    d. be accompanied by a female EMT if possible.

17. If an EMT elects to help an injured person and leaves him or her before other trained help arrives, the EMT may be sued for:

    a. dereliction.
    b. malfeasance.
    c. abandonment.
    d. lack of consent.

18. In most states, an individual is granted immunity from liability if he or she acts in good faith to provide care to his or her level of training and to the best of his or her ability. This protection is called:

    a. total patient protection.
    b. the good samaritan law.
    c. the duty to act.
    d. consent.

## SITUATIONS FOR FURTHER DISCUSSION

1. You arrive at the scene of a hit-and-run accident where a young child who was riding a bike is found unconscious. You initial survey indicates no overt signs of injury. The child's 16-year-old brother is also at the scene but was not involved in the accident. The injured child regains consciousness and claims not to be hurt. The older brother insists that you not treat the child. Both parents are at work.

   a. What do your primary and secondary surveys indicate the problem to be?

   b. What factors allow you to come to this conclusion?

   c. What factors caused you to rule out other conditions?

   d. What is the correct emergency treatment for this patient and in what order?

   e. In what position will you transport this patient?

   f. What continuing care will you provide for this patient en route to the hospital?

   g. What common allied problems might you expect to find or see develop with this patient's condition?

   h. What is the urgency of transportation to the hospital for this patient?

   i. What would be your radio report to the hospital regarding the situation and present condition of the patient?

2. You are dispatched to the scene of a two-car accident and find three victims. The driver of the first car, which has a star-burst pattern of broken glass on the windshield, is found unconscious, slumped over the wheel. The driver of the second car has a deep laceration of the upper arm which oozes a steady stream of blood. A child also is found who was knocked off his bike by one of the vehicles as it skidded. The child appears to have a fractured lower leg, vitals are stable, and the child's parents are not at the scene. The patient with the laceration appears coherent, has stable vitals, but refuses your care.

   a. What do your primary and secondary surveys indicate the problem to be?

   b. What factors allow you to come to this conclusion?

# 4 THE EMERGENCY MEDICAL TECHNICIAN

c. What factors caused you to rule out other conditions?

d. What is the correct emergency treatment for this patient and in what order?

e. In what position will you transport this patient?

f. What continuing care will you provide for this patient en route to the hospital?

g. What common allied problems might you expect to find or see develop with this patient's condition?

h. What is the urgency of transportation to the hospital for this patient?

i. What would be your radio report to the hospital regarding the situation and present condition of the patient?

# 2

# The Human Body

- *Overview of the Human Body*
- *Relating Structures to the Body*

---

1. The study of body function is called:
   a. anatomy.
   b. physiology. ✓
   c. embryology.
   d. histology.

2. The term used to describe movement away from the midline of the body is called:
   a. adduction.
   b. flexion.
   c. extension.
   d. abduction. ✓

3. When compared to the ankle, the knee is said to be:
   a. medial.
   b. distal.
   c. proximal. ✓
   d. lateral.

4. Dividing the body into right and left halves with a vertical line, anything away from the midline is said to be:
   a. proximal.
   b. distal.
   c. medial. ✓
   d. lateral. ✓

   medial | lateral
   proximal | distal

5. The term used to describe the front of the body is:
   a. superior.
   b. inferior.
   c. anterior. ✓
   d. posterior.

6. For quick reference, the abdomen is usually divided into:
   a. one quadrant.
   b. two quadrants.
   c. three quadrants.
   d. four quadrants. ✓

7. In reference to the stomach, the heart is:
   a. anterior. front
   b. posterior. back
   c. superior. ✓
   d. inferior. lower

8. The act of bending at a joint is called:
   a. flexion. ✓ flex
   b. extension. extend
   c. tension.
   d. adduction.

9. The lungs, heart, and great blood vessels are contained in the:
   a. posterior cavity.
   b. pelvic cavity.
   c. abdominopelvic cavity.
   d. thoracic cavity. ✓

10. The cranial and spinal cavities collectively comprise the:
    a. anterior cavity.
    b. posterior cavity. ✓
    c. ventral cavity.
    d. medial cavity.

## 6 THE HUMAN BODY

11. The body system that produces chemicals called hormones and helps regulate most body functions is called the:
    a. integumentary system.
    b. nervous system.
    c. reticuloendothelial system.
    d. endocrine system.

12. The network of specialized cells found within the connective tissues whose main function is to kill microorganisms is called the:
    a. immune system.
    b. endocrine system.
    c. integumentary system.
    d. musculoskeletal system.

13. The anterior body cavity below the diaphragm containing the digestive and reproductive organs is called the:
    a. stomach.
    b. right upper quadrant.
    c. abdominopelvic cavity.
    d. dorsal cavity.

14. A person lying on his or her left side is said to be in a:
    a. right recumbent position.
    b. left lateral recumbent position.
    c. left medial recumbent position.
    d. supine position.

15. The appendix and part of the large intestine are located in the:
    a. right upper quadrant.
    b. left upper quadrant.
    c. right lower quadrant.
    d. left lower quadrant.

16. The small hard spot just below the sternum is the:
    a. heart.
    b. suprasternal notch.
    c. gallbladder.
    d. xiphoid process.

17. The structure located below the liver is the:
    a. spleen.
    b. pancreas.
    c. gallbladder.
    d. duodenum.

18. The structure located lateral to the left side of the stomach is the:
    a. spleen.
    b. pancreas.
    c. gallbladder.
    d. duodenum.

19. Which of the following structures is located in all four abdominal quadrants?
    a. Liver.
    b. Kidneys.
    c. Large intestine.
    d. Diaphragm.

20. The movement to turn a hand or foot inward toward the midline is called:
    a. lateral rotation.
    b. medial rotation.
    c. abduction.
    d. adduction.

21. All of the following structures are considered to be within the abdominal cavity *except* the:
    a. duodenum.
    b. spleen.
    c. kidneys.
    d. appendix.

22. The term used to describe the lower jaw is the:
    a. mandible.
    b. maxilla.
    c. ilium.
    d. frontanel.

23. The term used to describe the base of the skull just above the neck is the:
    a. parietal region.
    b. zygomatic region.
    c. mastoid process.
    d. orbital region.

24. The bone on the medial aspect of the lower leg is called the:
    a. tibia.
    b. fibula.
    c. patella.
    d. femur.

25. The bone that arches over the urinary bladder is called the:

    a. iliac crest.
    b. costal arch.
    c. symphysis pubis. *(circled)*
    d. ilium.

26. At the proximal end of the femur is the:

    a. greater trochanter. *(circled)*
    b. patella.
    c. tibia.
    d. medial femoral condyle.

27. The ulnar shaft is:

    a. on the lateral aspect of the lower arm.
    b. on the medial aspect of the lower arm. *(circled)*
    c. attached to the humerus at the lateral humeral condyle.
    d. directly attached to the acromioclavicular joint.

28. The occipital bone is located:

    a. at the back of the skull. *(circled)*
    b. at the top of the skull.
    c. at the front of the skull.
    d. superior to the parietal bone.

29. With respect to the diaphragm, the lungs are:

    a. distal.
    b. proximal.
    c. superior. *(circled)*
    d. inferior.

30. Which of the following is considered to be a hollow structure?

    a. kidneys.
    b. pancreas.
    c. spleen.
    d. duodenum. *(circled)*

## SITUATIONS FOR FURTHER DISCUSSION

1. You are called to the home of a middle-aged woman who tripped and fell down a flight of stairs. She is found in a supine position with her head tilted toward the left side. Her left arm is flexed and her right arm is abducted. Both her legs appear laterally rotated. The patient is conscious and complains of extreme pain while trying to move.

   a. What do your primary and secondary surveys indicate the problem to be?

   *Pt fall from stairs, multiple fx, poss. C-spine*

   b. What factors allow you to come to this conclusion?

   *Arm flexed, arm abducted, legs lat rotated, extreme pain*

   c. What factors caused you to rule out other conditions?

   *extreme pain*

   d. What is the correct emergency treatment for this patient and in what order?

   *C-spine, airway, breathing, circ*

   e. In what position will you transport this patient?

   *Full C-spine poss*

   f. What continuing care will you provide for this patient en route to the hospital?

   *Airway O2, Breathing, poss signs of shock*

## 8 THE HUMAN BODY

g. What common allied problems might you expect to find or see develop with this patient's condition?

h. What is the urgency of transportation to the hospital for this patient?

i. What would be your radio report to the hospital regarding the situation and present condition of the patient?

2. Your patient complains of a sharp pain in the lower right quadrant and also is nauseous. His pulse is rapid and weak.

   a. What do your primary and secondary surveys indicate the problem to be?

   *c/o sharp pain*
   *E(R)q  Poss.*
   *LRQ, appendicitis*
   *nauseous*

   b. What factors allow you to come to this conclusion?

   *Location of pain, rapid pulse weak*
   *Sx shock*

   c. What factors caused you to rule out other conditions?

   d. What is the correct emergency treatment for this patient and in what order?

   *O2*

   e. In what position will you transport this patient?

   *Supine  Legs flexed elev*

   f. What continuing care will you provide for this patient en route to the hospital?

   *Monitor VS*
   *O2*

   g. What common allied problems might you expect to find or see develop with this patient's condition?

   h. What is the urgency of transportation to the hospital for this patient?

   *3*

   i. What would be your ratio report to the hospital regarding the situation and present condition of the patient?

   *Ringdown*
   *Hosp.*
   *unit NO.*
   *Sharp pain RLQ*
   *pt age*
   *pt gender*
   *tx.*
   *Sx shock  ETA*

3. A patient is found who has an apparent fracture to the distal portion of the left femur. The left leg appears to be rotated externally and foreshortened.

   a. What do your primary and secondary surveys indicate the problem to be?

   *back*
   *?? pelvis*
   *Fx Ⓛ Leg*

   b. What factors allow you to come to this conclusion?

   *Leg rotated externally & foreshortened*

   c. What factors caused you to rule out other conditions?

   d. What is the correct emergency treatment for this patient and in what order?

   *C-spine*
   *① O₂*

   e. In what position will you transport this patient?

   f. What continuing care will you provide for this patient en route to the hospital?

   g. What common allied problems might you expect to find or see develop with this patient's condition?

   h. What is the urgency of transportation to the hospital for this patient?

   i. What would be your radio report to the hospital regarding the situation and present condition of the patient?

# 3

# Patient Assessment

- *Obtaining Information*
- *The Field Assessment*

---

1. The systematic gathering of information to determine a patient's illness or injury is called:
   a. primary survey.
   b. symptomology.
   c. vital signs.
   d. patient assessment.

2. Information gathered from the dispatcher and from bystanders at the scene should:
   a. not be considered as factual accounts of what happened.
   b. lead you to a quick conclusion.
   c. be ignored.
   d. be considered, but not as the sole basis for any conclusion.

3. A police officer is the first trained person on the scene of a motor vehicle accident and initiates a survey and treatment. You must:
   a. tell him to go direct traffic.
   b. tactfully assume responsibility for the patient and redo the survey.
   c. take the first responder's word about findings of the patient assessment and immediately initiate treatment.
   d. return to your base station since you are not needed.

4. Patient assessment is a systematic procedure:
   a. always done in a step-by-step manner.
   b. not always done in a step-by-step manner.
   c. done by as many trained responders as possible.
   d. starting at the feet and working towards the head.

5. The portion of the patient assessment utilized to detect life-threatening problems is called the:
   a. primary survey.
   b. secondary survey.
   c. pulse check.
   d. field assessment.

6. During the primary survey, the patient should be checked for profuse bleeding by:
   a. quickly scanning the patient for blood stains.
   b. rolling the patient over to check the underside of the patient.
   c. This is not routinely done during the primary survey.
   d. carefully looking and feeling for evidence of hemorrhage.

7. Equipment necessary to detect blood pressure includes a stethoscope and:
   a. watch with a sweep second hand.
   b. sphygmomanometer.
   c. auscultator.
   d. diastolic meter.

8. While checking for the mechanism of injury during the initial scene survey, the EMT should:
   a. develop tunnel vision to zero in on the problem.
   b. spend a good deal of time checking the mechanism of injury before doing the primary survey.
   c. be certain that no danger still exists before going to the patient's side.
   d. take the blood pressure at the same time.

9. An EMT finds an unconscious victim lying in a prone position and cannot determine if he is breathing. The EMT should:

   a. use the log roll maneuver to move the patient to the supine position so the EMT can check for breathing.
   b. not move the patient at all.
   c. move the patient only after completion of the secondary survey, after spinal injury has been ruled out.
   d. skip the check for breathing since the patient is face down.

10. The order of the primary survey is:

    a. airway, breathing, circulation, profuse bleeding.
    b. airway, breathing, circulation.
    c. airway, responsiveness, breathing, circulation.
    d. responsiveness, airway, breathing, circulation, profuse bleeding.

11. The results of information obtained during the survey are recorded:

    a. after the crew returns to quarters, usually from memory.
    b. on a legal document called the "survey form" as they are found.
    c. on the patient's medical chart at the Emergency Department by the EMT.
    d. in the EMT's notebook, and are a matter of public record.

12. When you first approach the victim, it is important to:

    a. say you are an "EMT."
    b. give your name and identify yourself as an "Emergency Medical Technician."
    c. not waste time in idle conversation with the victim.
    d. immediately treat all injuries without wasting time to talk to the patient.

13. To check an apparently unconscious victim for responsiveness, the EMT should:

    a. look, listen, and feel for air exchange.
    b. slap the patient's face.
    c. shake the patient to see if he or she is asleep.
    d. gently tap the patient's shoulders and shout, "Are you okay?".

14. The EMT establishes if there is heart action and blood circulation in the unconscious adult patient during the primary survey by checking the:

    a. carotid pulse on the same side as the EMT.
    b. carotid pulse on the side opposite the EMT.
    c. radial pulse.
    d. femoral pulse.

15. The comprehensive hands-on, head-to-toe survey is called the:

    a. primary survey.
    b. subjective interview.
    c. objective examination.
    d. triage.

16. If a patient refuses your offer to help, the EMT should:

    a. force the patient to allow treatment.
    b. immediately leave.
    c. continue to talk to the patient quietly, offering reassurance.
    d. restrain the patient.

17. The field examination should:

    a. take about 10 to 15 minutes to complete.
    b. consist of the primary and secondary surveys.
    c. involve checking only the surrounding area for clues.
    d. only allow for the quick detection of life-threatening problems.

18. To open the airway of an unconscious patient with a suspected spinal injury, the EMT should:

    a. perform a head-tilt neck-lift maneuver.
    b. perform a head-tilt chin-lift maneuver.
    c. perform a jaw thrust maneuver.
    d. not open the airway due to possible movement of the spine.

19. If the patient is unconscious, the EMT may gather information for the subjective interview:

    a. by asking the patient.
    b. by checking medic alert identification.
    c. There is no way this can be done since the patient is unconscious.
    d. after the patient regains consciousness, usually in the emergency room.

20. In checking for signs of breathing, the EMT should remember that females typically evidence more pronounced movement at the:

    a. abdomen.
    b. diaphragm.
    c. chest.
    d. clavicles.

## 12  PATIENT ASSESSMENT

21. During the primary survey, the EMT need only be concerned with bleeding that:

    a. has left the patient's face and head covered with blood but has stopped.
    b. oozes from a laceration.
    c. spurts or flows freely.
    d. The EMT should not be concerned with any hemorrhage during the primary survey.

22. Before starting the secondary survey, the EMT should always:

    a. look over the patient's condition for signs of deterioration.
    b. check the blood pressure.
    c. determine the pulse rate and quality.
    d. wait until all necessary equipment is at hand.

23. Anything that the patient tells you is wrong is considered:

    a. a symptom.
    b. a sign.
    c. a vital sign.
    d. not relevant to the patient assessment.

24. A sign of caring for the sick and injured is to place the back of your hand on the patient's forehead. Not only may you reassure the patient, you also may:

    a. shield bright lights from his or her eyes.
    b. keep his or her hair out of the eyes.
    c. gain information about his or her skin temperature.
    d. be able to check for a stoma.

25. What the EMT sees, hears, feels, or smells when examining the patient is considered:

    a. a diagnostic sign.
    b. a symptom.
    c. a vital sign.
    d. of little importance.

26. The normal pulse rate for an adult at rest is approximately:

    a. 60 to 80 beats per minute.
    b. 50 to 90 beats per minute.
    c. 75 beats per minute.
    d. 70 to 80 beats per minute.

27. The EMT should consider it serious if a child from one to five years of age has a respiratory rate at rest that is above:

    a. 40 breaths per minute.
    b. 24 breaths per minute.
    c. 36 breaths per minute.
    d. 44 breaths per minute.

28. If the EMT encounters a patient who is lying down, he or she should:

    a. immediately get the patient on his or her feet to try to "walk it off."
    b. walk the patient to the ambulance to increase circulation.
    c. find out if the patient lay down, was knocked down, fell, or was thrown into that position.
    d. place the patient in a sitting position so the blood pressure can be taken.

29. The normal pulse rate at rest for children between five and twelve years of age should be:

    a. 60 to 80 beats per minute.
    b. 70 to 100 beats per minute.
    c. 60 to 100 beats per minute.
    d. 60 to 120 beats per minute.

30. The blood pressure is normally measured by placing the blood pressure cuff over the:

    a. radial artery.
    b. femoral artery.
    c. brachial artery.
    d. carotid artery.

31. Children from five to twelve years of age are considered in need of a physician's care when their respiratory rate is greater than:

    a. 24 breaths per minute.
    b. 30 breaths per minute.
    c. 36 breaths per minute.
    d. 20 breaths per minute.

32. It is important for the EMT to learn whether the patient's current problem has happened before or whether the patient has ever felt this way before, because:

    a. both injuries and illness can sometimes be attributed to a past medical condition.
    b. new problems are less serious than recurring problems.
    c. it is polite to appear concerned about the patient's past problems.
    d. it will indicate how long the patient has been healthy.

33. The patient interview should:

    a. be completed before the objective interview begins.
    b. be completed before the subjective interview begins.

c. take place at the same time as the physical examination.
d. take place after the subjective interview.

34. The normal pulse rate at rest for children between the ages of one and five years is:

    a. 60 to 80 beats per minute.
    b. 80 to 100 beats per minute.
    c. 80 to 120 beats per minute.
    d. 80 to 150 beats per minute.

35. The blood pressure measured when the lower left chamber of the heart is relaxed and refilling:

    a. is the systolic blood pressure.
    b. is the diastolic blood pressure.
    c. is the first number reported, as in "120 over 80."
    d. cannot be determined by a blood pressure reading.

36. The normal respiratory rate for an adult at rest is:

    a. 12 to 20 breaths per minute.
    b. 10 to 18 breaths per minute.
    c. 12 to 18 breaths per minute.
    d. 12 to 24 breaths per minute.

37. One isolated blood pressure reading is:

    a. always meaningless.
    b. diagnostically significant if it is unusually low.
    c. called auscultation.
    d. determined most accurately by the auscultation method.

38. When checking the patient's eyes, the EMT finds larger than normal pupils. The pupils are said to be:

    a. dilated.
    b. constricted.
    c. unequal.
    d. pinpoint.

39. The EMT finds a clear fluid in the ear canal of a patient suspected of suffering a head injury. This fluid probably is:

    a. water.
    b. cerebrospinal fluid.
    c. amniotic fluid.
    d. mucal fluid.

40. Normal adult diastolic blood pressures usually range between:

    a. 60 to 70 mmHg.
    b. 80 and 120 mmHg.
    c. 60 and 90 mmHg.
    d. 50 and 100 mmHg.

41. Hypertension is considered when a child between the ages of one and five has a blood pressure:

    a. above 120 systolic.
    b. below 70 systolic.
    c. below 70 diastolic.
    d. above 120 diastolic.

42. Hypotension is considered when a child between the ages of five and twelve has a blood pressure:

    a. below 90 diastolic.
    b. below 90 systolic.
    c. above 90 systolic.
    d. between 90 and 150 systolic.

43. When the EMT determines the blood pressure without using a stethoscope, this procedure is called:

    a. a cuffless blood pressure.
    b. carotid blood pressure.
    c. blood pressure by auscultation.
    d. blood pressure by palpation.

44. Hypotension exists when the blood pressure:

    a. drops below 90 systolic.
    b. shows a systolic drop and diastolic rise.
    c. is between 90 and 120 systolic.
    d. rises above 145/95.

45. During the blood pressure check by auscultation, the systolic blood pressure is read:

    a. when the needle begins to jump.
    b. when you hear the beginning of clicking or tapping sounds.
    c. when you hear the sounds turn dull or disappear.
    d. when the radial pulse is no longer felt.

46. The EMT determines that the patient's skin is hot and dry. This indicates:

    a. shock.
    b. a normal condition.
    c. excessive body heat.
    d. loss of body heat.

47. Unequal pupils may indicate:

    a. cardiac arrest.
    b. narcotics use.
    c. use of LSD.
    d. stroke.

## 14 PATIENT ASSESSMENT

**48.** During the secondary survey, the EMT should check for a stoma. This usually is located in the:

   a. neck.
   b. abdomen.
   c. groin area.
   d. chest.

**49.** If, during any part of the secondary survey, the EMT finds evidence of possible spinal damage, he or she should:

   a. immediately place the victim on a long spine board.
   b. ask the patient not to move and continue the survey.
   c. immediately have his or her partner provide temporary immobilization to the neck and back and then continue the survey.
   d. record this information and continue the survey.

**50.** The persistent erection of a male's penis often brought about by spinal injury is called:

   a. stoma.
   b. priapism.
   c. cerebrospinal erection.
   d. a symptom.

### SITUATIONS FOR FURTHER DISCUSSION

**1.** A 25-year-old male who was injured in an electrical accident is found lying on the ground when you arrive and is no longer in contact with the electrical source. His skin appears pale, pulse is rapid and weak, respirations are rapid and shallow. The patient's blood pressure is 90/60 mmHg, and the skin is cool and clammy. Your survey also indicates a burn mark on his right hand from the electrical contact.

   a. What do your primary and secondary surveys indicate the problem to be?

   b. What factors allow you to come to this conclusion?

   c. What factors caused you to rule out other conditions?

   d. What is the correct emergency treatment for this patient and in what order?

   e. In what position will you transport this patient?

   f. What continuing care will you provide for this patient en route to the hospital?

   g. What common allied problems might you expect to find or see develop with this patient's condition?

   h. What is the urgency of transportation to the hospital for this patient?

   i. What would be your radio report to the hospital regarding the situation and present condition of the patient?

# 4

# Basic Life Support I: The Airway and Pulmonary Resuscitation

- *The Respiratory System*
- *Respiratory Failure*
- *Pulmonary Resuscitation*
- *Airway Obstruction*

---

1. The process of breathing, which takes place when the muscles attached to the rib cage and diaphragm contract, is called:

    a. metabolism.
    b. inspiration.
    c. regulation.
    d. expiration.

2. For the conscious patient with a partial airway obstruction, the EMT should:

    a. deliver four back blows and four abdominal thrusts.
    b. deliver back blows only.
    c. have the patient cough.
    d. be prepared for vomiting.

3. The larynx contains the:

    a. pharynx.
    b. voicebox.
    c. trachea.
    d. bronchial tree.

4. Oxygen is provided for the cells, carbon dioxide is removed, and the acid-base balance of the blood is maintained through the process called:

    a. edema.
    b. breathing.
    c. hypoxia.
    d. diaphoresis.

5. If the patient with a complete airway obstruction is a conscious infant:

    a. apply only sharp back blows until the airway is cleared.
    b. alternate four back blows and four abdominal thrusts until the airway is cleared or the patient becomes unconscious.
    c. alternate four back blows and four chest thrusts until the airway is cleared or the patient becomes unconscious.
    d. attempt a blind finger sweep to remove the obstruction.

6. The process of breathing, which takes place when the diaphragm and muscles attached to the ribs relax, is called:

    a. expiration.
    b. inspiration.
    c. metabolism.
    d. regulation.

7. An unusual breathing sound often due to a foreign object, blood, or other fluids in the trachea is:

    a. wheezing.
    b. crowing.
    c. gurgling.
    d. snoring.

8. Once the EMT is breathing for the patient, he or she must continue to do so:

   a. until the patient starts to vomit.
   b. until he or she transfers the responsibility to another trained responder.
   c. until he or she detects cardiac arrest.
   d. until gastric distention occurs.

9. Occasionally, the EMT will not be able to ventilate a nonbreathing patient with the standard technique due to severe injuries to the mouth, lower jaw, the patient's lack of teeth or dentures, or a receding chin. To ventilate these patients:

   a. use the jaw thrust maneuver.
   b. There is no special technique; proceed as usual.
   c. use mouth-to-nose ventilations.
   d. use a modified head tilt.

10. Swelling due to excessive fluid in the tissues is called:

    a. edema.
    b. pleura.
    c. cyanosis.
    d. dyspnea.

11. Which of the following may cause a full or partial upper airway obstruction?

    a. Congestive heart failure
    b. A deviated septum
    c. Breathing hot air, as in a fire
    d. Chronic obstructive pulmonary disease

12. Which of these unusual breathing sounds is most likely caused by the tongue obstructing the pharynx?

    a. Wheezing
    b. Crowing
    c. Gurgling
    d. Snoring

13. The ideal rate for mouth-to-mouth ventilations for infants is one gentle breath every:

    a. 3 seconds.
    b. 5 seconds.
    c. 7 seconds.
    d. 10 seconds.

14. When breathing stops completely, the patient is in:

    a. cardiac arrest.
    b. respiratory arrest.
    c. clinical death.
    d. biological death.

15. The distress signal for choking usually displayed by conscious victims of complete airway obstruction is:

    a. clutching the neck between thumb and fingers.
    b. coughing.
    c. speaking in a low voice.
    d. patting themselves on the back.

16. Once gastric distention begins, the EMT should:

    a. try to reposition the head to provide a better airway.
    b. discontinue breaths if vomiting occurs.
    c. deliver breaths at a rate of five per minute.
    d. deliver abdominal thrusts.

17. The major muscle used in breathing is the:

    a. heart.
    b. lungs.
    c. diaphragm.
    d. larynx.

18. The trachea is also known as the:

    a. adam's apple.
    b. epiglottis.
    c. windpipe.
    d. pharynx.

19. If the EMT's first attempt to ventilate an unconscious, nonbreathing patient is not successful, he or she should:

    a. deliver four back blows.
    b. check the carotid pulse.
    c. alternate four back blows and four manual thrusts.
    d. reposition the head and attempt to ventilate again.

20. Crowing is an unusual breathing sound that may indicate a partial airway obstruction, probably caused by:

    a. the tongue.
    b. fluids in the trachea.
    c. spasms of the larynx.
    d. a foreign object in the trachea.

21. To open the airway of an infant or small child:

    a. a slight head tilt will not be adequate.
    b. hyperextend adequately.
    c. do not hyperextend the neck.
    d. use the jaw thrust maneuver as a first resort.

22. A laryngectomy patient breathes through:

    a. the nose.
    b. the mouth.
    c. a stoma.
    d. an S-tube.

23. In cases where a patient has an apparent partial airway obstruction but cannot cough or has a very weak cough, the EMT should:

    a. wait until the patient becomes unconscious before beginning treatment.
    b. treat the patient as if there is a complete airway obstruction.
    c. keep the patient's head turned to the side.
    d. insert an airway.

24. Clinical death occurs:

    a. with the death of the patient's brain cells.
    b. 10 minutes after biological death.
    c. the moment breathing stops and the heart stops beating.
    d. only to patients suffering myocardial infarctions.

25. When the patient is in respiratory arrest, the EMT should use:

    a. cardiopulmonary resuscitation.
    b. mouth-to-mouth ventilation.
    c. direct pressure.
    d. a nasal cannula.

26. When the EMT uses the mouth-to-mouth technique on an adult patient, breaths must be delivered to the patient once every:

    a. 5 seconds.
    b. 3 seconds.
    c. 10 seconds.
    d. 15 seconds.

27. How many times per minute is the process of breathing repeated in the average adult male at rest?

    a. 10 to 18
    b. 12 to 20
    c. 15 to 25
    d. 10 to 24

28. Each breath taken by an average adult male moves approximately:

    a. 1 liter or 1000 cc of air.
    b. ½ liter or 500 cc of air.
    c. 2 liters or 2000 cc of air.
    d. 1½ liters or 1500 cc of air.

29. When an EMT performs mouth-to-mouth ventilations, the air provided for the nonbreathing patient contains:

    a. 16 percent oxygen.
    b. 21 percent oxygen.
    c. 6 percent oxygen.
    d. 10 percent oxygen.

30. The pharynx is also referred to as the:

    a. throat.
    b. voicebox.
    c. windpipe.
    d. adam's apple.

31. A large, double-layered membranous sac lines the thoracic cavity and covers the outside of the lungs. This sac is the:

    a. bronchial sac.
    b. laryngeal membrane.
    c. pleura.
    d. pericardium.

32. The thoracic cavity is separated from the abdomino-pelvic cavity by the:

    a. lungs.
    b. diaphragm.
    c. heart.
    d. pericardium.

33. When a patient is in respiratory arrest, he or she is:

    a. no longer pulsing.
    b. no longer breathing.
    c. in need of cardiopulmonary rescuscitation.
    d. clinically dead.

34. Signs of adequate breathing may include:

    a. no chest movement, no air felt or heard at the nose or mouth, and cyanosis.
    b. uneven chest movement, noisy breathing, rapid respiratory rate, very deep or labored breathing.
    c. air exchange evaluated as below normal, slow rate of respirations, shallow breathing.
    d. even chest movement, air felt or heard at the nose or mouth.

35. Biological death occurs:

    a. the moment breathing stops and the heart stops.
    b. with the death of brain cells.
    c. when the patient suffers a cerebral vascular accident.
    d. 10 minutes before clinical death.

## 18  BASIC LIFE SUPPORT I: THE AIRWAY AND PULMONARY RESUSCITATION

36. The only widely recommended procedure for opening the airway of unconscious patients with possible neck or spinal injuries is the:

    a. head-tilt maneuver.
    b. head-tilt, chin-lift maneuver.
    c. head-tilt, neck-lift maneuver.
    d. jaw thrust maneuver.

37. Many problems of partial airway obstruction, particularly those caused by the tongue, can be corrected by:

    a. opening the airway.
    b. providing four rapid, full thrusts.
    c. finger sweeps.
    d. providing four manual thrusts.

38. The "trapdoor-like" structure that normally prevents food, liquids, and foreign objects from entering the airway is the:

    a. epiglottis.
    b. tongue.
    c. pharynx.
    d. thyroid cartilage.

39. Within the lungs, the exchange of oxygen and carbon dioxide takes place in the:

    a. bronchioles.
    b. alveoli.
    c. bronchi.
    d. capillaries.

40. The condition where the patient's skin, lips, earlobes, or nailbeds turn blue or gray due to a lack of oxygen in circulation is called:

    a. cyanosis.
    b. rigor mortis.
    c. dyspnea.
    d. edema.

41. A common occurrence when a patient's head flexes forward and is allowed to remain in that position is:

    a. edema of the airway.
    b. airway obstruction by the pharynx.
    c. dyspnea.
    d. airway obstruction by the tongue.

## SITUATIONS FOR FURTHER DISCUSSION

1. You respond to a call involving a woman choking at a restaurant. When you arrive the woman appears cyanotic, is clutching her throat, and cannot talk. The patient also appears to be seven or eight months pregnant.

    a. What do your primary and secondary surveys indicate the problem to be?

    b. What factors allow you to come to this conclusion?

    c. What factors caused you to rule out other conditions?

    d. What is the correct emergency treatment for this patient and in what order?

    e. In what position will you transport this patient?

    f. What continuing care will you provide for this patient en route to the hospital?

BASIC LIFE SUPPORT I: THE AIRWAY AND PULMONARY RESUSCITATION   19

g. What common allied problems might you expect to find or see develop with this patient's condition?

h. What is the urgency of transportation to the hospital for this patient?

i. What would be your radio report to the hospital regarding the situation and present condition of the patient?

2. You arrive at the scene and find a young child unconscious and cyanotic. The child is lying next to his mother's handbag, and there are several coins scattered about him. Further inspection indicates that he is not breathing and nothing is visible inside the mouth.

   a. What do your primary and secondary surveys indicate the problem to be?

   b. What factors allow you to come to this conclusion?

   c. What factors caused you to rule out other conditions?

d. What is the correct emergency treatment for this patient and in what order?

e. In what position will you transport this patient?

f. What continuing care will you provide for this patient en route to the hospital?

g. What common allied problems might you expect to find or see develop with this patient's condition?

h. What is the urgency of transportation to the hospital for this patient?

i. What would be your radio report to the hospital regarding the situation and present condition of the patient?

# 5

# Basic Life Support II: CPR - Cardiopulmonary Resuscitation

- *The Heart*
- *CPR*

---

1. The pulse measured by palpating the major artery of the upper arm is the:

    a. radial.
    b. femoral.
    c. brachial.
    d. mediastinal.

2. The greatest enemies of a healthy body include all of these EXCEPT:

    a. lack of exercise.
    b. stress.
    c. jogging or aerobic exercise.
    d. poor diet.

3. CPR is indicated:

    a. when a patient's heart and lung actions have stopped.
    b. to every patient suffering a heart attack.
    c. to any collapsed victim.
    d. only to heart attack victims.

4. The ABCs of emergency care stand for:

    a. Airway, Bleeding, Circulation.
    b. Adequate Body Compression.
    c. Airway, Breathing, Circulation.
    d. Administer Basic CPR.

5. The cardiac arrest victim should be placed:

    a. on a hard surface.
    b. in the prone position.
    c. with the upper extremities elevated.
    d. directly on the ambulance cot.

6. How deep should the chest of an adult be compressed during CPR?

    a. 1½ to 2 inches
    b. 1½ to 2½ inches
    c. 1 to 2 inches
    d. ¾ to 1½ inches

7. Clinical death occurs:

    a. 10 minutes after biological death.
    b. when heart beat and respirations stop.
    c. when irreversible brain damage has occurred.
    d. 10 minutes after cardiac arrest.

8. Artificial circulation is produced when the heart is compressed between the:

    a. sternum and diaphragm.
    b. ribs and spine.
    c. sternum and spine.
    d. xiphoid process and spine.

9. What is the most common complication when performing chest compressions during CPR?

   a. Injury to the rib cage
   b. Vomiting
   c. Rigormortis
   d. Obstructed airway

10. The EMT can determine that chest compressions are effective:

    a. if cyanosis develops.
    b. if a pulse is felt during compressions.
    c. if the pupils dilate.
    d. The EMT cannot determine this in the field.

11. If there is no one on hand to help when you discover a patient in cardiac arrest, you should:

    a. phone immediately for help, then provide CPR.
    b. perform CPR without stopping until someone who can help comes, or you become exhausted.
    c. perform CPR for one minute, phone for help, then return to providing CPR.
    d. perform CPR for at least five minutes, then go for help.

12. Once CPR has been instituted, it must be continued until:

    a. the victim develops a spontaneous pulse.
    b. 20 minutes have elapsed without change.
    c. rigormortis is detected.
    d. cyanosis becomes pronounced.

13. The breathing check on an unresponsive victim is performed:

    a. immediately.
    b. after the pulse check.
    c. after delivering 2 breaths.
    d. after establishing an open airway.

14. During one-rescuer CPR, compressions are delivered at a rate of:

    a. 80–100 per minute.
    b. 60–80 per minute.
    c. 100–120 per minute.
    d. 40–60 per minute.

15. Blood is sent to the lungs to be oxygenated from the:

    a. left atrium.
    b. left ventricle.
    c. right atrium.
    d. right ventricle.

16. The central portion of the thoracic cavity, containing the heart, its greater blood vessels, part of the trachea, and part of the esophagus, is called the:

    a. pericardium.
    b. mediastinum.
    c. sternum.
    d. diaphragm.

17. The membraneous sac that surrounds the heart is called the:

    a. diaphragm.
    b. ventricle.
    c. pericardium.
    d. mediastinum.

18. The transportation of blood from the right side of the heart to the lungs is called:

    a. systemic circulation.
    b. pulmonary circulation.
    c. coronary circulation.
    d. cerebral circulation.

19. The aorta begins the:

    a. systemic circulation.
    b. pulmonary circulation.
    c. coronary circulation.
    d. cerebral circulation.

20. During one-rescuer CPR, how many compressions are delivered in one minute?

    a. 60
    b. 80
    c. 120
    d. 100

21. What is the ratio of compressions to ventilations for one-rescuer CPR?

    a. 15 to 2
    b. 5 to 1
    c. 15 to 1
    d. 5 to 2

22. During CPR, when should the pulse of the victim be checked?

    a. After the first minute and every few minutes thereafter
    b. Every minute
    c. After 5 minutes and every 10 minutes thereafter
    d. Every 2 minutes

## 22  BASIC LIFE SUPPORT II: CPR

23. Cardiopulmonary Resuscitation (CPR) is:

    a. artificial respiration.
    b. heart resuscitation.
    c. the treatment for all heart attacks.
    d. heart-lung resuscitation.

24. Cardiac arrest occurs when the:

    a. victim suffers a heart attack.
    b. pulse is weak and thready.
    c. heart suffers reduced output.
    d. heart stops beating, no longer circulating blood.

25. The proper CPR compression site on an adult is:

    a. approximately one finger-width superior to the substernal notch.
    b. midsternum.
    c. on the small projection at the inferior end of the sternum.
    d. approximately one finger-width inferior to the suprasternal notch.

26. To determine if CPR is needed for an infant, the EMT should check the:

    a. carotid pulse.
    b. apical pulse.
    c. brachial pulse.
    d. radial pulse.

27. The xiphoid process is:

    a. the bone to which the ribs attach.
    b. the CPR compression site.
    c. a small projection at the inferior end of the sternum.
    d. a general term for the uppermost region on the sternum to which the ribs attach.

28. The substernal notch is:

    a. the CPR compression site.
    b. a general term for the lowest region on the sternum to which the ribs attach.
    c. where the clavicles meet the sternum.
    d. another term for the xiphoid process.

29. In opening the airway of an infant or small child, use the head-tilt, chin-lift technique and apply:

    a. a standard tilt.
    b. an extra-exaggerated tilt.
    c. a slight tilt.
    d. a jaw thrust.

30. A CPR victim is considered an infant from:

    a. birth to 3 months.
    b. 3 months to 6 months.
    c. birth to 2 years.
    d. birth to 1 year.

31. During CPR on a child, the rate of compressions is:

    a. 60–80 per minute.
    b. 80–100 per minute.
    c. 100–120 per minute.
    d. 120–140 per minute.

32. The flat bone located on the anterior of the chest, that connects the ribs and is the site for CPR compressions, is called the:

    a. xiphoid process.
    b. sternum.
    c. mediastinum.
    d. rib cage.

33. Biological death occurs:

    a. at the moment breathing and heart beat cease.
    b. only in cases of terminal, irreversible illness.
    c. when a physician pronounces the victim to be dead.
    d. when the victim's brain cells begin to die.

34. You will maintain an open airway, supply breaths, and force the victim's heart to circulate blood during:

    a. rescue breathing.
    b. CPR.
    c. a blood pressure check.
    d. the obstructed airway maneuver.

35. During infant CPR, the infant's sternum should be compressed:

    a. ¼ to ¾ inch.
    b. ½ to ¾ inch.
    c. ½ to 1 inch.
    d. ¼ to 1 inch.

36. To perform CPR on an infant, use the:

    a. heel of one hand.
    b. thumbs.
    c. tips of two or three fingers.
    d. heels of two hands.

37. What is the correct ratio of compressions to ventilations for CPR on a child?

    a. 15 to 2
    b. 5 to 1
    c. 15 to 1
    d. 5 to 2

38. The CPR compression site on children is:

    a. on the small projection at the inferior end of the sternum.
    b. approximately three finger-widths superior to the suprasternal notch.
    c. midsternum, directly between the nipples.
    d. the same as for an adult.

39. In providing ventilations to an infant, the rescuer should provide:

    a. a full breath in order to totally expand the victim's lungs.
    b. a small puff, being careful not to expand the lungs.
    c. a gentle breath, enough to cause the infant's chest to rise.
    d. a large, oversized breath.

40. What is the correct ratio of compressions to ventilations for infant CPR?

    a. 15 to 2
    b. 5 to 1
    c. 15 to 1
    d. 5 to 2

41. To perform CPR on a child, use the:

    a. heel of one hand.
    b. thumbs.
    c. tips of two or three fingers.
    d. heels of two hands.

42. During infant CPR, what is the rate of compressions?

    a. 60 per minute
    b. 80 per minute
    c. 100 per minute
    d. 120 per minute

43. A CPR victim is considered a child from:

    a. 2 years to 12 years.
    b. 3 months to 10 years.
    c. 1 year to 8 years.
    d. 3 years to 10 years.

44. An advantage of two-rescuer CPR is:

    a. the victim requires less oxygen.
    b. compressions are not interrupted.
    c. fewer compressions are required per minute.
    d. the victim receives more oxygen.

45. During two-rescuer CPR, what is the rate of compressions?

    a. 40–60 per minute
    b. 60–80 per minute
    c. 80–100 per minute
    d. 100–120 per minute

46. What is the correct ratio of compressions to ventilations in two-rescuer CPR?

    a. 15 to 2
    b. 5 to 1
    c. 15 to 1
    d. 5 to 2

47. If during two-rescuer CPR, the rescuer misses a breath, he or she should:

    a. wait for the next fifth upstroke.
    b. have the compressor go back and count the fifth compression again.
    c. deliver the breath on the upstroke of the next compression.
    d. let the compressor wait until the breath is delivered.

48. During two-rescuer CPR, the ventilator delivers a full breath during the:

    a. downstroke of the fifth compression.
    b. downstroke of the fifteenth compression.
    c. upstroke of the fifth compression.
    d. upstroke of the fifteenth compression.

49. The compressor counts out loud saying, "One, and; two, and; three, and; . . . during:

    a. one-rescuer CPR.
    b. two-rescuer CPR.
    c. both one- and two-rescuer CPR.
    d. infant CPR.

50. During two-rescuer CPR, the change is controlled by the:

    a. compressor.
    b. ventilator.
    c. crew chief.
    d. patient.

## BASIC LIFE SUPPORT II: CPR

51. During the two-rescuer change, it is recommended that the carotid pulse and breathing be checked by:
    a. the ventilator before moving to the chest.
    b. the compressor as he moves to the ventilator position.
    c. by both the ventilator and compressor together.
    d. it is not necessary to check the pulse during two-rescuer CPR.

52. During CPR on a child, the sternum should be compressed:
    a. 1 to 1½ inches.
    b. ½ to 1 inch.
    c. ¾ to 1½ inches.
    d. ½ to ¾ inch.

53. The major blood vessel leading from the heart to the body, which has a one-way valve to keep blood from leaking back into the left ventricle, is the:
    a. pulmonary artery.
    b. aorta.
    c. atrium.
    d. coronary artery.

54. The type of circulation in which blood is pumped from the heart to the lungs and then back to the heart is called:
    a. coronary circulation.
    b. pulmonary circulation.
    c. systemic circulation.
    d. thoracic circulation.

55. The type of circulation in which blood is pumped from the heart, out to the entire body, and back to the heart is called:
    a. coronary circulation.
    b. pulmonary circulation.
    c. systemic circulation.
    d. thoracic circulation.

56. The tubular structure leading from the throat to the stomach is the:
    a. trachea.
    b. epiglottis.
    c. esophagus.
    d. thorax.

57. When the heel of the hand is placed over the CPR compression point, the fingers should be:
    a. curved between the ribs.
    b. curled into a fist.
    c. off the chest.
    d. pressing downward.

58. The reason for using four to ten seconds to establish unresponsiveness in a collapsed victim is:
    a. the victim may only have fainted.
    b. it helps to increase unnecessary resuscitation.
    c. it may prevent possible damage to the xiphoid process.
    d. to allow time to bare the chest.

59. The EMT can determine if an unconscious victim is breathing by:
    a. checking the blood pressure.
    b. checking the cyanosis at the lips and nail beds.
    c. checking the pulse and pupils.
    d. looking, listening, and feeling for signs of air and chest movement.

60. Complications that may result from cardiac compressions, even when correctly performed, include:
    a. xiphoid process depressed into liver.
    b. fractured collar bone.
    c. fractured ribs.
    d. collapsed trachea.

61. The heel of the hand should stay in contact with the chest during compressions because:
    a. chest expansion with respirations will be easier to feel.
    b. correct position can be maintained.
    c. slapping against the chest wall will cause more heart damage.
    d. gastric distention is minimized.

62. If you begin two-rescuer CPR with the assistance of a bystander and find that the volunteer is unable to perform CPR correctly, you should:
    a. stop CPR just long enough to offer brief training.
    b. insist that the volunteer move to the head to deliver breaths.
    c. stop the two-rescuer CPR and begin one-rescuer CPR.
    d. count out loud, coaching the volunteer in the proper procedure.

63. The beating of the heart is an automatic, involuntary process. The heart has its own pacemaker and a system of specialized muscle tissues that allow the heart to beat. This is called the:

    a. nerve impulse system.
    b. conduction system.
    c. regulatory system.
    d. heart control system.

64. What condition should exist before the EMT attempts to revive a victim by performing CPR?

    a. Permanent brain damage has occurred.
    b. Evidence that breathing and the pulse are absent.
    c. The victim's pupils are dilated.
    d. The victim has shallow respirations.

65. CPR should not be interrupted unnecessarily; maximum interruption should not exceed:

    a. 10 seconds for any reason.
    b. 10 seconds for intubation.
    c. 10 seconds during stairway transportation.
    d. 7 seconds with specific exceptions.

66. One circumstance under which CPR may be discontinued is:

    a. when the EMT thinks the victim will not survive.
    b. when the EMT suspects the victim will suffer permanent brain damage.
    c. when the EMT is exhausted and unable to continue.
    d. when the EMT sees no reaction of the pupils or other signs of life.

67. Which of the following is the best indication that external chest compressions are producing adequate blood flow?

    a. Change in patient's color.
    b. Constriction of the pupils.
    c. A second rescuer feels a pulse in the carotid artery with each compression.
    d. There is no way to determine this without special instruments.

68. How much time may be taken initially to make sure the individual does not have a pulse?

    a. 10 seconds
    b. 12 seconds
    c. 15 seconds
    d. 20 seconds

69. Since successful resuscitation of drowning victims has been reported after prolonged periods of submersion in cold water, the EMT should:

    a. leave drowning victims in the water for as long as possible.
    b. initiate CPR even if the victim has been submerged for 20 to 30 minutes, or more.
    c. delay CPR because of the hypothermia effect.
    d. use the back-pressure, arm-lift method of resuscitation.

70. To determine whether an adult victim has a pulse, the EMT should palpate the pulse at the:

    a. carotid artery in the neck.
    b. femoral artery in the groin.
    c. brachial artery in the arm.
    d. radial artery in the wrist.

71. How many ventilations are provided to an infant victim during one minute of CPR?

    a. 10
    b. 12
    c. 20
    d. 24

72. When two EMTs are performing CPR, the EMT giving chest compressions:

    a. should pause after every fifth compression while the second EMT gives ventilations.
    b. should pause after every twelfth compression while the second EMT gives ventilations.
    c. should not pause while the second EMT interposes ventilations during the upstroke of each fifth compression.
    d. should not pause after compressions unless he or she becomes tired.

73. During external chest compression, if the hands are placed too low on the sternum:

    a. the collar bone may be fractured.
    b. the lungs may be lacerated.
    c. the liver may be lacerated.
    d. the heart may be bruised.

74. If the patient has numerous rib fractures, a flail chest, a neck injury or has recently had heart surgery, external cardiac compressions for a pulseless victim are:

    a. too hazardous to perform.
    b. never too hazardous to perform.
    c. require a physician's approval.
    d. to be performed only by a physician.

## 26  BASIC LIFE SUPPORT II: CPR

**75.** When the patient bleeds profusely during CPR, the EMT must:

   a. apply a tourniquet, treat for shock, and not resume CPR.
   b. apply a tourniquet and discontinue CPR.
   c. treat for shock.
   d. correct the bleeding and then continue CPR.

**76.** Oxygenated blood is pumped to the body from the:

   a. right atrium.
   b. right ventricle.
   c. left atrium.
   d. left ventricle.

**77.** During the compression phase of CPR, blood is pumped:

   a. only through the systematic circulation.
   b. only through the pulmonary circulation.
   c. through both the systemic and pulmonary circulations.
   d. only through major organs.

**78.** Even when CPR is performed correctly ribs may be fractured. In such cases the EMT should:

   a. stop CPR to prevent further damage.
   b. stop compressions, continue ventilations.
   c. not stop CPR, but reassess hand location.
   d. change places with his or her partner.

**79.** The EMT can determine circulation on a child by palpating the:

   a. radial pulse.
   b. carotid pulse.
   c. brachial pulse.
   d. apical pulse.

**80.** As an EMT, be certain to practice CPR on infant and adult mannikins. You must be recertified in CPR:

   a. at least once a year.
   b. at least once every two years.
   c. only if you do not practice regularly.
   d. An EMT does not need to become recertified.

## SITUATIONS FOR FURTHER DISCUSSION

**1.** You find a 40-year-old male lying in bed who has gone into cardiac arrest. There is no prior history of cardiac problems in the patient, according to family members. The wife initiated mouth-to-mouth resuscitation 10 minutes ago, but no cardiac compressions have been given.

   a. What do your primary and secondary surveys indicate the problem to be?

   b. What factors allow you to come to this conclusion?

   c. What factors caused you to rule out other conditions?

   d. What is the correct emergency treatment for this patient and in what order?

   e. In what position will you transport this patient?

   f. What continuing care will you provide for this patient en route to the hospital?

g. What common allied problems might you expect to find or see develop with this patient's condition?

h. What is the urgency of transportation to the hospital for this patient?

i. What would be your radio report to the hospital regarding the situation and present condition of the patient?

2. You respond to find an elderly woman in cardiac arrest who is located on the third floor of an apartment building that has no elevator. A neighbor who knows CPR was present when the woman went into arrest and immediately started CPR.

   a. What do your primary and secondary surveys indicate the problem to be?

   b. What factors allow you to come to this conclusion?

   c. What factors caused you to rule out other conditions?

d. What is the correct emergency treatment for this patient and in what order?

e. In what position will you transport this patient?

f. What continuing care will you provide for this patient en route to the hospital?

g. What common allied problems might you expect to find or see develop with this patient's condition?

h. What is the urgency of transportation to the hospital for this patient?

i. What would be your radio report to the hospital regarding the situation and present condition of the patient?

## 28  BASIC LIFE SUPPORT II: CPR

3. You are at a family picnic and a small child is lost. A short time later, someone finds the child at the bottom of a pool next door. Upon removing the child from the water, you detect no respirations and no pulse. The nearest ambulance service is located 20 miles away in the next town.

   a. What do your primary and secondary surveys indicate the problem to be?

   b. What factors allow you to come to this conclusion?

   c. What factors caused you to rule out other conditions?

   d. What is the correct emergency treatment for this patient and in what order?

   e. In what position will you transport this patient?

   f. What continuing care will you provide for this patient en route to the hospital?

   g. What common allied problems might you expect to find or see develop with this patient's condition?

   h. What is the urgency of transportation to the hospital for this patient?

   i. What would be your radio report to the hospital regarding the situation and present condition of the patient?

4. You respond to a local nursing home for an elderly man who has gone into cardiac arrest. During compressions, you feel ribs crack under your compressions.

   a. What do your primary and secondary surveys indicate the problem to be?

   b. What factors allow you to come to this conclusion?

   c. What factors caused you to rule out other conditions?

# BASIC LIFE SUPPORT II: CPR

d. What is the correct emergency treatment for this patient and in what order?

e. In what position will you transport this patient?

f. What continuing care will you provide for this patient en route to the hospital?

g. What common allied problems might you expect to find or see develop with this patient's condition?

h. What is the urgency of transportation to the hospital for this patient?

i. What would be your radio report to the hospital regarding the situation and present condition of the patient?

5. While performing CPR on a 50-year-old male in a restaurant, you notice that the abdomen appears distended.

a. What do your primary and secondary surveys indicate the problem to be?

b. What factors allow you to come to this conclusion?

c. What factors caused you to rule out other conditions?

d. What is the correct emergency treatment for this patient and in what order?

e. In what position will you transport this patient?

f. What continuing care will you provide for this patient en route to the hospital?

g. What common allied problems might you expect to find or see develop with this patient's condition?

h. What is the urgency of transportation to the hospital for this patient?

i. What would be your radio report to the hospital regarding the situation and present condition of the patient?

# 6

# Breathing Aids and Oxygen Therapy

- *Aids to Breathing*
- *Oxygen Therapy*

---

1. Oropharyngeal airways can be used on a patient if:

    a. the patient gives you verbal permission.
    b. a physician orders it regardless of the patient's level of consciousness.
    c. the patient is unconscious and has no gag reflex.
    d. the patient is a neck breather.

2. The nonbreathing patient should be suctioned for no more than:

    a. 15 seconds before attempting to provide two ventilations.
    b. 10 seconds before attempting to provide two ventilations.
    c. 5 seconds before attempting to provide two ventilations.
    d. 30 seconds or until all fluids have been cleared from the airway.

3. The facepiece used with a demand-valve resuscitator or bag-valve-mask resuscitator should:

    a. be of rigid design.
    b. have perforations in the sides for exhaled air.
    c. be clear to allow seeing vomitus.
    d. contain an outlet port for exhaled air.

4. The term atelectasis describes:

    a. air sac collapse.
    b. infant eye damage due to high concentrations of oxygen.
    c. a side effect of COPD.
    d. hemoglobin insufficiency.

5. When the EMT inserts the oropharyngeal airway, it should be inserted:

    a. straight into place, curved side down.
    b. sideways and rotated a quarter turn.
    c. upside down and rotated 180 degrees when it is clear of the tongue.
    d. curved side up and rotated 90 degrees when it is clear of the tongue.

6. The most common problem encountered when using a bag-valve-mask resuscitator is:

    a. the bag refills slowly.
    b. several EMTs are required to use the device.
    c. the delivery valve freezes.
    d. an improper seal between the face and mask.

7. The maximum concentration of oxygen that should be administered to a COPD patient who is not suffering respiratory or cardiac arrest is:

    a. 2 percent.
    b. 16 percent.
    c. 21 percent.
    d. 28 percent.

## 32 BREATHING AIDS AND OXYGEN THERAPY

8. A Bourdon gauge flowmeter is:
   a. a single-stage pressure regulator.
   b. fairly inaccurate at low flow rates.
   c. accurate at all flow rates.
   d. gravity dependent.

9. The proper size oropharyngeal airway should fit with the flange:
   a. just below the teeth.
   b. just above the teeth, but below the lips.
   c. just above the lips.
   d. just below the base of the tongue.

10. Atmospheric air provides what percentage of oxygen to the patient who is breathing spontaneously?
    a. 4 percent
    b. 16 percent
    c. 21 percent
    d. 100 percent

11. The term used to describe a decrease in the supply of oxygen in the body tissues is:
    a. hypoxia.
    b. anoxia.
    c. atelectasis.
    d. oxygen toxicity.

12. Positive pressure ventilation describes when the EMT:
    a. uses pressurized oxygen cylinders.
    b. utilizes a device to force oxygen into the patient's lungs.
    c. uses a venturi mask.
    d. uses a pressure-compensated flowmeter.

13. If the EMT inserts an oropharyngeal airway that is too long for the size of the patient's oropharynx:
    a. the airway may be swallowed by the patient.
    b. it will not be possible to insert an airway that is too long.
    c. the excess length can extend outside the lips without causing any problems.
    d. it may push the tongue back into the pharynx.

14. During bag-mask resuscitation of a nonbreathing adult patient, the EMT should squeeze the bag-valve-mask resuscitator every:
    a. 3 seconds.
    b. 5 seconds.
    c. 10 seconds.
    d. 12 seconds.

15. When premature infants are administered too much oxygen, scar tissue can form behind the lens of the eye. This is called:
    a. anoxia.
    b. atelectasis.
    c. retrolental fibroplasia.
    d. oxygen toxicity.

16. The EMT must switch to a fresh oxygen cylinder when the gauge reaches the safe residual pressure of:
    a. 200 PSI.
    b. 200 LPM.
    c. zero pressure.
    d. the patient cannot get any more oxygen with each breath.

17. The suction catheter should not be inserted too deeply into the oropharynx so as to induce the gag reflex. The EMT can measure the proper length of the suction catheter by:
    a. measuring the catheter from the corner of the jaw to the corner of the mouth.
    b. inserting the catheter to the point at which the patient gags.
    c. inserting until the black mark on the catheter is at the lips.
    d. measuring the catheter from the center of the mouth to the angle of the jaw.

18. The effective concentration of oxygen delivered to a patient using an oxygen-enriched pocket mask with an oxygen flow rate of 10 LPM is:
    a. 16 percent oxygen.
    b. 21 percent oxygen.
    c. 45 percent oxygen.
    d. 98 percent oxygen.

19. The COPD patient has, over a period of time, developed an increase in blood carbon dioxide. The primary center for respiration no longer responds to high carbon dioxide levels in the blood. Respiratory control is taken over by secondary centers located in the:
    a. carotid arteries.
    b. brain.
    c. heart.
    d. lungs.

20. Mouth-to-mouth resuscitation delivers:
    a. 98 percent oxygen to the patient.
    b. 21 percent oxygen to the patient.
    c. 16 percent oxygen to the patient.
    d. 4 percent oxygen to the patient.

21. Hemoglobin insufficiency is a cause of:
    a. oxygen toxicity.
    b. infant eye damage.
    c. alveolar collapse.
    d. hypoxia.

22. A full portable D cylinder contains:
    a. 500 liters of oxygen.
    b. 350 liters of oxygen.
    c. 625 liters of oxygen.
    d. 2000 liters of oxygen.

23. The type of oxygen flowmeter capable of indicating the actual flow at all times is the:
    a. pressure-compensated flowmeter.
    b. Bourdon gauge flowmeter.
    c. humidified type.
    d. Bourdon gauge flowmeter with humidifier.

24. The proper size oropharyngeal airway can be determined by measuring from the:
    a. center of the mouth to the angle of the jaw.
    b. nose to the earlobe.
    c. nose to the angle of the jaw.
    d. corner of the mouth to the angle of the jaw.

25. Approximately how long may the EMT expect to be able to use an M cylinder if the gauge initially reads 1800 PSI and the flow rate will be set at 10 LPM?
    a. 1 hour
    b. 3 hours
    c. 4.5 hours
    d. 6 hours

26. A nasal cannula used with oxygen at a flow rate of 2 LPM will deliver oxygen to the patient at a concentration of:
    a. 2 percent.
    b. 28 percent.
    c. 40 percent.
    d. 100 percent.

27. A venturi mask with a flow rate of 4 LPM will deliver oxygen at a concentration of 24 percent. The same mask at 8 LPM will deliver what concentration of oxygen?
    a. 24 percent
    b. 48 percent
    c. 40 percent
    d. 28 percent

28. Resuscitation using the bag-valve-mask resuscitator without any oxygen adjuncts provides what percentage oxygen to the patient?
    a. 24 percent
    b. 16 percent
    c. 21 percent
    d. 40 percent

29. The oxygen delivery device of choice for use by the EMT on COPD patients is the:
    a. nasal cannula.
    b. simple face mask.
    c. partial rebreathing bag.
    d. venturi mask.

30. During one-rescuer CPR, the best resuscitation method for the EMT to use is:
    a. mouth-to-mouth resuscitation.
    b. a pocket mask with adjunct oxygen.
    c. a bag-valve-mask resuscitator.
    d. a venturi mask.

31. Which of the following delivers the highest concentration of oxygen to the nonbreathing patient?
    a. the pocket mask
    b. the bag-valve-mask resuscitator
    c. the venturi mask
    d. the demand valve resuscitator

32. If an unconscious patient develops a gag reflex while an oropharyngeal airway is inserted into the oropharynx, the EMT should:
    a. push the airway back into place.
    b. remove the airway, clean it off, and replace it.
    c. remove the airway at once.
    d. remove the airway, suction the oropharynx, and reinsert the airway.

33. Hypoxic hypoxia is a term used to describe:
    a. cellular exchange problems.
    b. hemoglobin insufficiency.
    c. circulatory insufficiency.
    d. respiratory insufficiency.

34. The simple face mask when used with a flow rate of 6 to 15 LPM will deliver an effective oxygen concentration to the patient from 35 percent to:
    a. 40 percent.
    b. 50 percent.
    c. 60 percent.
    d. 100 percent.

## 34 BREATHING AIDS AND OXYGEN THERAPY

35. The minimum flow rate that can be used with the non-rebreathing face mask is:

    a. 2 LPM.
    b. 8 LPM.
    c. 15 LPM.
    d. 30 LPM.

36. If hypoxia is allowed to continue untreated, the patient will:

    a. develop respiratory arrest.
    b. suffer alveolar collapse.
    c. develop oxygen toxicity.
    d. develop COPD.

37. Carbon dioxide can build up within the simple face mask if the flow rate is set below:

    a. 6 LPM.
    b. 8 LPM.
    c. 10 LPM.
    d. 12 LPM.

38. A pressure regulator is used to reduce the pressure in an oxygen cylinder to a safe working pressure of:

    a. 30 to 70 PSI.
    b. 15 LPM.
    c. 50 to 100 PSI.
    d. 2000 PSI.

39. The maximum flow rate to be used with a nasal cannula is:

    a. 6 LPM.
    b. 10 LPM.
    c. 15 LPM.
    d. 30 LPM.

40. The partial rebreathing face mask when used at a flow rate between 6 and 10 LPM will deliver oxygen from:

    a. 20 to 50 percent.
    b. 35 to 60 percent.
    c. 30 to 70 percent.
    d. 50 to 98 percent.

## SITUATIONS FOR FURTHER DISCUSSION

1. You must transfer a patient from the local hospital to another hospital which is located three hours away. The patient is a cardiac patient currently breathing with supplemental oxygen through a face mask at 8 liters per minute. The ambulance contains a "G" size tank that shows 1200 psi.

    a. What do your primary and secondary surveys indicate the problem to be?

    b. What factors allow you to come to this conclusion?

    c. What factors caused you to rule out other conditions?

    d. What is the correct emergency treatment for this patient and in what order?

    e. In what position will you transport this patient?

    f. What continuing care will you provide for this patient en route to the hospital?

g. What common allied problems might you expect to find or see develop with this patient's condition?

h. What is the urgency of transportation to the hospital for this patient?

i. What would be your radio report to the hospital regarding the situation and present condition of the patient?

2. You respond to a home and find a male who is not breathing but still has a strong carotid pulse. Your initial attempts to ventilate are met by resistance, but further inspection shows that this patient is a neck breather. What oxygen adjuncts would you use to treat this patient?

   a. What do your primary and secondary surveys indicate the problem to be?

   b. What factors allow you to come to this conclusion?

   c. What factors caused you to rule out other conditions?

d. What is the correct emergency treatment for this patient and in what order?

e. In what position will you transport this patient?

f. What continuing care will you provide for this patient en route to the hospital?

g. What common allied problems might you expect to find or see develop with this patient's condition?

h. What is the urgency of transportation to the hospital for this patient?

i. What would be your radio report to the hospital regarding the situation and present condition of the patient?

# 36 BREATHING AIDS AND OXYGEN THERAPY

3. You have just delivered a patient to the emergency room who required suctioning during transportation. What must you do to ready the equipment before you put the ambulance back in service?

   a. What do your primary and secondary surveys indicate the problem to be?

   b. What factors allow you to come to this conclusion?

   c. What factors caused you to rule out other conditions?

   d. What is the correct emergency treatment for this patient and in what order?

   e. In what position will you transport this patient?

   f. What continuing care will you provide for this patient en route to the hospital?

   g. What common allied problems might you expect to find or see develop with this patient's condition?

   h. What is the urgency of transportation to the hospital for this patient?

   i. What would be your radio report to the hospital regarding the situation and present condition of the patient?

4. You must transport a COPD patient to the hospital. During transportation, what device would you use to administer oxygen and at what flow rate?

   a. What do your primary and secondary surveys indicate the problem to be?

   b. What factors allow you to come to this conclusion?

   c. What factors caused you to rule out other conditions?

BREATHING AIDS AND OXYGEN THERAPY  37

d. What is the correct emergency treatment for this patient and in what order?

e. In what position will you transport this patient?

f. What continuing care will you provide for this patient en route to the hospital?

g. What common allied problems might you expect to find or see develop with this patient's condition?

h. What is the urgency of transportation to the hospital for this patient?

i. What would be your radio report to the hospital regarding the situation and present condition of the patient?

# 7

# Basic Life Support III: Bleeding and Shock

## SECTION ONE: BASIC PROCEDURES

- *Bleeding*
- *Shock*

---

1. The watery, salty fluid that makes up over half the volume of the blood is:
   a. white blood cells.
   b. plasma.
   c. platelets.
   d. red blood cells.

2. The pressure point used to control profuse bleeding from the knee is the:
   a. femoral.
   b. pedal.
   c. subclavian.
   d. radial.

3. Treatment for shock is included in emergency care procedures for:
   a. only those who request it.
   b. only those who are unconscious.
   c. every serious injury and medical problem.
   d. only those whose blood pressure is below 100/70.

4. Shock caused by blood loss is called:
   a. septic shock.
   b. hypovolemic shock.
   c. cardiogenic shock.
   d. metabolic shock.

5. Care of a patient in shock includes:
   a. control bleeding, avoid rough handling, administer fluids orally, keep the patient lying still.
   b. administer oxygen, position the patient to elevate the lower extremities regardless of fractures, monitor the vital signs.
   c. assure an adequate airway and breathing, splint fractures, give nothing by mouth, prevent loss of body heat.
   d. administer oxygen, place the patient in a sitting position, monitor vital signs, and keep warm.

6. A condition often brought about by fear, bad news, the sight of blood, or a minor injury is:
   a. anaphylactic shock.
   b. respiratory shock.
   c. septic shock.
   d. psychogenic shock.

7. Dark maroon blood flowing steadily from the wound indicates:
   a. venous bleeding.
   b. capillary bleeding.
   c. bronchiole bleeding.
   d. arterial bleeding.

8. Once you have applied a tourniquet:
   a. loosen only if it is painful for the patient.
   b. leave it in place. Do not loosen.
   c. loosen every twenty minutes.
   d. loosen every ten minutes.

9. The EMT should consider that internal bleeding is severe if the patient:
   a. experience abdominal tenderness.
   b. is vomiting blood that looks like coffee grounds.
   c. has a slow, full pulse.
   d. is unconscious.

10. Of the following types of shock, which is considered to be self-correcting?
    a. Metabolic
    b. Respiratory
    c. Neurogenic
    d. Psychogenic

11. As a result of bleeding from major neck veins:
    a. pressure points cannot be used as a means of controlling bleeding.
    b. the patient may require radiation therapy as a result of the injury.
    c. air may be sucked in and form an air embolism that can be carried to the heart.
    d. a tourniquet must be used to control the bleeding.

12. Which type of shock occurs when a person contacts something to which he or she is extremely allergic?
    a. Respiratory shock
    b. Anaphylactic shock
    c. Metabolic shock
    d. Cardiogenic shock

13. Direct pressure held firmly on a wound will usually stop mild bleeding in:
    a. 1 to 2 minutes.
    b. 1 to 10 minutes.
    c. 10 to 30 minutes.
    d. 30 to 40 minutes.

14. Which "formed" elements of the blood release chemical factors needed to form blood clots when ruptured?
    a. White blood cells
    b. Plasma
    c. Platelets
    d. Red blood cells

15. Metabolic shock is also known as:
    a. lung shock.
    b. body fluid shock.
    c. allergy shock.
    d. bloodstream shock.

16. When providing care for a patient with possible internal bleeding, what should be your first concern?
    a. Keep the patient lying down and at rest.
    b. Maintain an open airway.
    c. Monitor vital signs.
    d. Reassure the patient.

17. What type of shock is caused by loss of plasma, as seen with burns or crushing injuries?
    a. Septic shock
    b. Hypovolemic shock
    c. Cardiogenic shock
    d. Respiratory shock

18. A marked drop in the blood pressure to 90 over 60 or lower is a sign of:
    a. shock.
    b. fractured skull.
    c. anxiety.
    d. coma.

19. The "Vial of Life" sticker on a patient's refrigerator is a sign that:
    a. the patient is an organ donor.
    b. patient information and medication can be found inside the refrigerator.
    c. the patient is a blood donor.
    d. the patient is a member of a safety patrol.

20. The signs of shock can include:
    a. rapid, weak pulse; deep, slow breathing; pale, moist skin.
    b. restlessness; pale, moist, cool skin; constricted pupils.
    c. rapid, weak pulse; rapid, shallow respirations; marked drop in blood pressure.
    d. rapid, bounding pulse; deep respirations; hot, moist skin.

21. A minimum blood loss that the EMT must consider to be life threatening to an adult is:
    a. 4 liters.
    b. 3 liters.
    c. 2 liters.
    d. 1 liter.

22. The typical adult male has approximately:
    a. 5 liters of blood.
    b. 12 liters of blood.
    c. 10 liters of blood.
    d. 4 liters of blood.

23. Shock caused by severe infection is called:
    a. septic shock.
    b. anaphylactic shock.
    c. metabolic shock.
    d. respiratory shock.

24. To estimate internal blood loss, assume that for every deep bruise found on the chest or abdomen the size of a man's fist, that the amount of blood lost is:
    a. 2 percent.
    b. 5 percent.
    c. 10 percent.
    d. 15 percent.

25. Shock may develop if blood volume is lost, blood vessels dilate to create a vascular capacity too great to be filled by the available blood, or:
    a. blood vessels constrict.
    b. the blood is over-oxygenated.
    c. there is intracranial hemorrhage.
    d. the heart fails as a pump.

26. Signs of anaphylactic shock can include:
    a. rapid, strong pulse.
    b. elevated blood pressure.
    c. headache and occasional loss of memory.
    d. marked swelling of the face and tongue, often with cyanosis of the lips.

27. Anaphylactic shock is a:
    a. true emergency requiring immediate medical care.
    b. low priority emergency.
    c. situation requiring slow and careful transport.
    d. self-correcting form of shock.

28. The "formed" elements of the blood whose primary function is to carry oxygen to the tissues and carry carbon dioxide away from the tissues are called:
    a. white blood cells.
    b. plasma.
    c. platelets.
    d. red blood cells.

29. Pressure over which artery can be used to control profuse bleeding of the forearm?
    a. Radial artery
    b. Carotid artery
    c. Brachial artery
    d. Subclavian artery

30. Shock is defined as:
    a. the failure of the cardiovascular system to provide sufficient blood circulation to all parts of the body.
    b. a result of blood vessels constricting and dilating to keep the circulatory system filled with blood.
    c. a quickening of the body processes.
    d. a loss of 5 percent or more of blood volume.

31. Of the following types of shock, which is caused by failure of the heart to pump blood adequately to all parts of the body?
    a. Hemorrhagic or hypovolemic shock
    b. Psychogenic shock
    c. Cardiogenic shock
    d. Metabolic shock

32. The procedure used only as a last resort, when all other methods have failed to control life-threatening bleeding from an extremity, is:
    a. the tourniquet.
    b. the pressure point.
    c. elevation.
    d. the inflatable airsplint.

33. When a dressing becomes blood soaked, the EMT should:
    a. remove the soaked dressing, and replace it with a sterile dressing.
    b. remove the soaked dressing to check the wound and blood flow.
    c. apply another dressing on top of the blood-soaked dressing and hold them both in place.
    d. use a pressure point to control the bleeding.

34. If bleeding is profuse, the EMT should:
    a. not waste time trying to find a dressing.
    b. use only a sterile dressing.
    c. immediately apply a tourniquet.
    d. use only a sterile bandage.

35. When the EMT applies a tourniquet, he should:
    a. select material that is between ¼ and 1 inch wide.
    b. attach a notation to the patient indicating that a tourniquet has been applied and the time of application.
    c. place the tourniquet as close to the torso as possible.
    d. continue to tighten the tourniquet, even after the bleeding stops.

36. Shock caused by the failure of the nervous system to control the diameter of blood vessels is:
    a. metabolic shock.
    b. cardiogenic shock.
    c. hypovolemic or hemorrhagic shock.
    d. neurogenic shock.

37. Bright red blood spurting from a wound indicates:
    a. arterial bleeding.
    b. venous bleeding.
    c. capillary bleeding.
    d. pneumatic bleeding.

38. The most effective method of controlling external bleeding is use of:
    a. pressure points.
    b. elevation.
    c. tourniquets.
    d. direct pressure.

39. The formed elements of the blood involved in destroying microorganisms and producing antibodies that help the body resist infection are:
    a. white blood cells.
    b. plasma.
    c. platelets.
    d. red blood cells.

40. The patient in shock usually will have:
    a. unequal pupils.
    b. constricted pupils.
    c. dilated pupils.
    d. restricted pupils.

41. Which form of shock is a temporary condition and considered self-correcting?
    a. Psychogenic shock
    b. Respiratory shock
    c. Anaphylactic shock
    d. Septic shock

42. Which of the following is the life-threatening reaction of the body to an allergic reaction?
    a. Respiratory shock
    b. Anaphylactic shock
    c. Septic shock
    d. Psychogenic shock

43. Pressure over which artery is used by the EMT to control profuse bleeding from some areas of the scalp?
    a. Facial artery
    b. Temporal artery
    c. Carotid artery
    d. Subclavian artery

## SITUATIONS FOR FURTHER DISCUSSION

1. The frantic mother of a child who put his hand through a storm door window has applied a tourniquet before you arrive to control the bleeding. The child is conscious, alert, pulse is rapid and strong, respirations are normal, and skin color and temperature are normal. There are no further signs of hemorrhage. When you question the mother, she tells you that the blood was flowing steadily from the laceration so she placed a tourniquet on the child's arm.

    a. What do your primary and secondary surveys indicate the problem to be?

    b. What factors allow you to come to this conclusion?

    c. What factors caused you to rule out other conditions?

**42** BASIC LIFE SUPPORT III: BLEEDING AND SHOCK SECTION ONE

d. What is the correct emergency treatment for this patient and in what order?

e. In what position will you transport this patient?

f. What continuing care will you provide for this patient en route to the hospital?

g. What common allied problems might you expect to find or see develop with this patient's condition?

h. What is the urgency of transportation to the hospital for this patient?

i. What would be your radio report to the hospital regarding the situation and present condition of the patient?

2. You are called to treat a child on the baseball field who feels dizzy, nauseous, and has a swollen face. His breathing appears labored, the pulse is thready, and the blood pressure is 90/60 mmHg.

a. What do your primary and secondary surveys indicate the problem to be?

b. What factors allow you to come to this conclusion?

c. What factors caused you to rule out other conditions?

d. What is the correct emergency treatment for this patient and in what order?

e. In what position will you transport this patient?

f. What continuing care will you provide for this patient en route to the hospital?

g. What common allied problems might you expect to find or see develop with this patient's condition?

h. What is the urgency of transportation to the hospital for this patient?

i. What would be your radio report to the hospital regarding the situation and present condition of the patient?

3. You respond to treat a fainting victim who has been revived before you arrive. The patient now refuses your assistance.

   a. What do your primary and secondary surveys indicate the problem to be?

   b. What factors allow you to come to this conclusion?

   c. What factors caused you to rule out other conditions?

d. What is the correct emergency treatment for this patient and in what order?

e. In what position will you transport this patient?

f. What continuing care will you provide for this patient en route to the hospital?

g. What common allied problems might you expect to find or see develop with this patient's condition?

h. What is the urgency of transportation to the hospital for this patient?

i. What would be your radio report to the hospital regarding the situation and present condition of the patient?

# 44 BASIC LIFE SUPPORT III: BLEEDING AND SHOCK SECTION ONE

4. Your patient was involved in a motorcycle accident and suffered a possible fractured femur. He now appears cyanotic, the skin is cool and clammy, and the pulse is rapid and weak. No other injuries are evident.

   a. What do your primary and secondary surveys indicate the problem to be?

   b. What factors allow you to come to this conclusion?

   c. What factors caused you to rule out other conditions?

   d. What is the correct emergency treatment for this patient and in what order?

   e. In what position will you transport this patient?

   f. What continuing care will you provide for this patient en route to the hospital?

   g. What common allied problems might you expect to find or see develop with this patient's condition?

   h. What is the urgency of transportation to the hospital for this patient?

   i. What would be your radio report to the hospital regarding the situation and present condition of the patient?

# 7

# Basic Life Support III: Bleeding and Shock

## SECTION TWO: PNEUMATIC COUNTERPRESSURE DEVICES—THE ANTI-SHOCK GARMENT

- *Anti-Shock Garments*

---

1. The anti-shock garment is used primarily for the patient who has developed or is certain to develop severe:

   a. metabolic shock.
   b. septic shock.
   c. hypovolemic shock.
   d. hypervolemic shock.

2. The use of the anti-shock garment is indicated for patients with a systolic blood pressure less than:

   a. 110 mmHg.
   b. 100 mmHg.
   c. 90 mmHg.
   d. 80 mmHg.

3. Anti-shock garments are contraindicated for patients suffering:

   a. pelvic fractures.
   b. pulmonary edema.
   c. fractures of the femur.
   d. pregnancy with indications of shock.

4. When placing a patient in the anti-shock garment, the patient should be placed:

   a. with the upper edge of the garment below the rib cage.
   b. with the upper edge of the garment above the rib cage.
   c. face down.
   d. on his or her side.

5. When inflating the anti-shock garment, the EMT should inflate the:

   a. abdomen section first.
   b. right leg section first.
   c. left leg section first.
   d. both leg sections first.

6. When inflating the anti-shock garment, the EMT should pump until:

   a. the gauge indicates 200 mmHg.
   b. air exhausts through the relief valves.
   c. the patient's blood pressure reaches 130 mmHg.
   d. the velcro straps release.

7. The EMT may remove the anti-shock garment when:
   a. the patient's color returns.
   b. the patient's blood pressure reaches 120 systolic.
   c. the patient's blood pressure reaches 80 diastolic.
   d. a physician orders the garment removed.

**46**  BASIC LIFE SUPPORT III: BLEEDING AND SHOCK  SECTION TWO

8. To deflate the anti-shock garment, the EMT should deflate:

   a. the abdominal section first.
   b. the leg sections first.
   c. all three sections slowly at once.
   d. all three sections rapidly at once.

### SITUATIONS FOR FURTHER DISCUSSION

1. You respond to treat a victim who is suffering a gunshot wound to the right thigh. The patient has lost a large amount of blood and has a blood pressure of 70/40 mmHg.

   a. What do your primary and secondary surveys indicate the problem to be?

   b. What factors allow you to come to this conclusion?

   c. What factors caused you to rule out other conditions?

   d. What is the correct emergency treatment for this patient and in what order?

   e. In what position will you transport this patient?

   f. What continuing care will you provide for this patient en route to the hospital?

   g. What common allied problems might you expect to find or see develop with this patient's condition?

   h. What is the urgency of transportation to the hospital for this patient?

   i. What would be your radio report to the hospital regarding the situation and present condition of the patient?

2. Your patient was involved in a motorcycle accident and suffered a possible fractured femur. She now appears cyanotic, the skin is cool and clammy, and the pulse is rapid and weak. The patient appears to be 7 months pregnant.

   a. What do your primary and secondary surveys indicate the problem to be?

   b. What factors allow you to come to this conclusion?

c. What factors caused you to rule out other conditions?

d. What is the correct emergency treatment for this patient and in what order?

e. In what position will you transport this patient?

f. What continuing care will you provide for this patient en route to the hospital?

g. What common allied problems might you expect to find or see develop with this patient's condition?

h. What is the urgency of transportation to the hospital for this patient?

i. What would be your radio report to the hospital regarding the situation and present condition of the patient?

3. A man is treated who has suffered a massive laceration to the leg with a significant loss of blood. He exhibits audible rales and has a blood pressure of 80/40 mmHg.

   a. What do your primary and secondary surveys indicate the problem to be?

   b. What factors allow you to come to this conclusion?

   c. What factors caused you to rule out other conditions?

   d. What is the correct emergency treatment for this patient and in what order?

   e. In what position will you transport this patient?

   f. What continuing care will you provide for this patient en route to the hospital?

## 48 BASIC LIFE SUPPORT III: BLEEDING AND SHOCK SECTION TWO

g. What common allied problems might you expect to find or see develop with this patient's condition?

h. What is the urgency of transportation to the hospital for this patient?

i. What would be your radio report to the hospital regarding the situation and present condition of the patient?

# 8

# Injuries I: Soft Tissues and Internal Organs

- *The Soft Tissues*
- *Types of Soft Tissue Injury*
- *Soft Tissue Wound Care*

---

1. The outermost layer of the skin is the:
   a. dermis.
   b. epidermis.
   c. subcutaneous layer.
   d. subdural.

2. A smooth cut made by a sharp object, such as a razor blade, is called:
   a. an incision.
   b. a laceration.
   c. an avulsion.
   d. an abrasion.

3. When an extremity is completely cut through or torn off, it is called:
   a. an avulsion.
   b. an amputation.
   c. an incision.
   d. a laceration.

4. The material used to hold sterile material over a wound:
   a. must be sterile.
   b. must be adhesive.
   c. is a dressing.
   d. is a bandage.

5. Clothing that covers a soft tissue injury:
   a. must be left in place.
   b. should be removed in the usual manner.
   c. should be removed only by the triage nurse.
   d. must be lifted, cut or split away.

6. In cases where open wounds of the abdomen are so large and deep that organs protrude through the wound opening, the EMT should:
   a. try to replace the protruding organ.
   b. cover the organ and wound opening.
   c. place ice packs on the wound to keep it cool.
   d. avoid administering oxygen.

7. The skin, muscles, blood vessels, nerves, fatty tissues, and tissues that line or cover organs are:
   a. soft tissues.
   b. hard tissues.
   c. cartilage tissues.
   d. connective tissues.

8. Skinned elbows and knees, "mat burns," "rug burns," and "brush burns" are examples of:
   a. hematomas.
   b. avulsions.
   c. lacerations.
   d. abrasions.

9. When the tip of the nose is cut or torn off, or an eye is pulled from its socket, the wound is an:
   a. avulsion.
   b. amputation.
   c. incision.
   d. abrasion.

10. Any material applied directly to a wound in an effort to control bleeding and prevent further contamination:
    a. is a bandage.
    b. is a dressing.
    c. should not be sterile.
    d. should be loosely secured to facilitate rapid inspection.

11. The layer of skin rich in blood vessels, nerves, and specialized structures such as sweat glands and hair follicles is the:
    a. epidermis.
    b. subdural layer.
    c. dermis.
    d. subcutaneous layer.

12. Of the following, which applies to general bandaging?
    a. All dressings should be bandaged very tightly in place to restrict blood flow.
    b. The ends of gauze, tape, or cloth bandages should be left loose to facilitate later removal.
    c. When bandaging extremities, leave the tips of the fingers and toes exposed whenever possible.
    d. Remove blood-soaked dressings and replace with clean dressings.

13. When caring for a patient with an object impaled in the abdomen, the EMT should:
    a. remove the impaled object and control bleeding.
    b. leave clothing in place so as not to move the object.
    c. stabilize the impaled object and control bleeding.
    d. place the patient in a sitting position to place pressure on the abdominal organs.

14. A closed wound is:
    a. an avulsion.
    b. an incision.
    c. an abrasion.
    d. a hematoma.

15. Both an entrance wound and an exit wound are present with which injury?
    a. An incision
    b. A penetrating puncture wound
    c. A laceration
    d. A perforating puncture wound

16. Swelling and deformity at the site of a bruise should alert the EMT to possible:
    a. contusions.
    b. abrasions.
    c. edema.
    d. underlying fractures.

17. Which type of wound has a jagged cut in which the tissues are snagged and torn, forming a rough edge around the wound?
    a. An incision
    b. A laceration
    c. A contusion
    d. A hematoma

18. Which of the following is an occlusive dressing?
    a. Nonadhering gauze roller
    b. Adhering gauze roller
    c. Petroleum gel-impregnated gauze
    d. Butterfly

19. Use of a sterile dressing on an open would will:
    a. reduce further contamination.
    b. kill any bacteria present in the wound.
    c. only be necessary if the wound is bleeding profusely.
    d. prevent shock.

20. To ensure control of bleeding and adequate wound care for a gunshot wound, the EMT must:
    a. apply a tourniquet immediately.
    b. search for an exit wound.
    c. leave the wound exposed; do not cover it.
    d. pack the wound with sterile gauze.

21. The most common form of closed wound is:
    a. an abrasion.
    b. a contusion.
    c. a laceration.
    d. an incision.

22. After a dressing has been applied to a wound, if bleeding continues, the EMT should:
    a. remove the blood-soaked dressing and replace it with clean, sterile dressings.
    b. leave the original dressing in place and place new dressings over the blood-soaked ones.
    c. bandage the dressing in place, even if the bleeding is not controlled.

d. lift the dressing only long enough to ascertain the severity of the continued bleeding.

23. When caring for an avulsed part which has been torn off, the EMT should:

   a. save the avulsed part in sterile saline solution and keep it as cold as possible.
   b. save the avulsed part by laying it directly on a bed of ice.
   c. wrap the avulsed part in a dry sterile dressing and put it in a plastic bag and keep it as cool as possible.
   d. place the avulsed part in its normal position and bandage it in place.

24. A blood clot almost always forms at the site of a contusion. The process taking place as blood seeps into the surrounding tissues to form a black-and-blue mark is called:

   a. epistaxis.
   b. edema.
   c. ecchymosis.
   d. alkalosis.

25. If the EMT believes there are internal injuries, the EMT should:

   a. assist the patient in taking sips of salted water.
   b. apply a cervical collar and place the patient on a long spine board.
   c. treat as if there is hemorrhage—treat for shock.
   d. apply a pressure bandage to the abdomen.

26. The method of choice for the EMT to control bleeding from an amputation is:

   a. the tourniquet.
   b. elevation.
   c. the snug pressure dressing.
   d. the loose sterile dressing.

27. The butterfly bandage may be used by the EMT to stabilize:

   a. minor lacerations.
   b. hematomas.
   c. sucking chest wounds.
   d. avulsions.

28. Which type of wound is caused by sharp, pointed objects such as nails, ice picks, splinters, or knives?

   a. Abrasion
   b. Avulsion
   c. Puncture
   d. Contusion

29. When it is necessary to form an airtight seal, the EMT should use:

   a. an occlusive dressing.
   b. sterile gauze pads.
   c. multitrauma or universal dressings.
   d. nonadhering gauze roller bandages.

30. Simple bruises, internal lacerations, and the rupturing of internal organs are called:

   a. closed wounds.
   b. open wounds.
   c. hard tissue injuries.
   d. medial injuries.

## SITUATIONS FOR FURTHER DISCUSSION

1. You are called to the scene of a stabbing. The victim is a 30-year-old male who is found lying on his side with a knife impaled in his chest just under the right nipple. A sucking sound is heard during respiration and the victim appears slightly cyanotic. The pulse is rapid, yet strong. No other injuries are found.

   a. What do your primary and secondary surveys indicate the problem to be?

   b. What factors allow you to come to this conclusion?

   c. What factors caused you to rule out other conditions?

   d. What is the correct emergency treatment for this patient and in what order?

**52** INJURIES I: SOFT TISSUES AND INTERNAL ORGANS

    e. In what position will you transport this patient?

    f. What continuing care will you provide for this patient en route to the hospital?

    g. What common allied problems might you expect to find or see develop with this patient's condition?

    h. What is the urgency of transportation to the hospital for this patient?

    i. What would be your radio report to the hospital regarding the situation and present condition of the patient?

2. While performing a survey on a patient who fell through a plate glass window, you encounter an avulsed flap of skin on the patient's back. The only other injuries you find are numerous small lacerations on the extremities which are bleeding very little. The patient does not appear cyanotic, and the vitals are normal, although the patient is in a great deal of pain.

    a. What do your primary and secondary surveys indicate the problem to be?

    b. What factors allow you to come to this conclusion?

    c. What factors caused you to rule out other conditions?

    d. What is the correct emergency treatment for this patient and in what order?

    e. In what position will you transport this patient?

    f. What continuing care will you provide for this patient en route to the hospital?

    g. What common allied problems might you expect to find or see develop with this patient's condition?

    h. What is the urgency of transportation to the hospital for this patient?

INJURIES I: SOFT TISSUES AND INTERNAL ORGANS   53

i. What would be your radio report to the hospital regarding the situation and present condition of the patient?

3. You are called to treat a 50-year-old man who fell while carrying a glass storm door and is found lying on his back with a bloodsoaked shirt in the abdominal area. The patient appears cyanotic, the pulse is rapid and weak, blood pressure is 100/70 mmHg. Your survey indicates a lacerated abdomen with several loops of bowel protruding through the laceration. Bleeding at the laceration site is not severe.

   a. What do your primary and secondary surveys indicate the problem to be?

   b. What factors allow you to come to this conclusion?

   c. What factors caused you to rule out other conditions?

   d. What is the correct emergency treatment for this patient and in what order?

   e. In what position will you transport this patient?

   f. What continuing care will you provide for this patient en route to the hospital?

   g. What common allied problems might you expect to find or see develop with this patient's condition?

   h. What is the urgency of transportation to the hospital for this patient?

   i. What would be your radio report to the hospital regarding the situation and present condition of the patient?

4. You are called to the scene of a bad car accident and find a patient who appears cyanotic and who has a pulse that is rapid and weak. Your survey indicates that his right leg has been amputated just above the knee. Bleeding from the wound appears heavy, but it is not spurting.

   a. What do your primary and secondary surveys indicate the problem to be?

   b. What factors allow you to come to this conclusion?

**54** INJURIES I: SOFT TISSUES AND INTERNAL ORGANS

    c. What factors caused you to rule out other conditions?

    d. What is the correct emergency treatment for this patient and in what order?

    e. In what position will you transport this patient?

    f. What continuing care will you provide for this patient en route to the hospital?

    g. What common allied problems might you expect to find or see develop with this patient's condition?

    h. What is the urgency of transportation to the hospital for this patient?

    i. What would be your radio report to the hospital regarding the situation and present condition of the patient?

**5.** During the physical assessment of a victim who was struck by a car while crossing the street, you find a bruise on the upper right quadrant of the patient's abdomen. The patient is semiconscious, and cyanotic, and the pulse is rapid and weak. No other injuries are found.

    a. What do your primary and secondary surveys indicate the problem to be?

    b. What factors allow you to come to this conclusion?

    c. What factors caused you to rule out other conditions?

    d. What is the correct emergency treatment for this patient and in what order?

    e. In what position will you transport this patient?

    f. What continuing care will you provide for this patient en route to the hospital?

# INJURIES I: SOFT TISSUES AND INTERNAL ORGANS

g. What common allied problems might you expect to find or see develop with this patient's condition?

h. What is the urgency of transportation to the hospital for this patient?

i. What would be your radio report to the hospital regarding the situation and present condition of the patient?

6. During treatment to a gunshot victim's chest wound, you notice a pool of blood developing from under the victim's back.

   a. What do your primary and secondary surveys indicate the problem to be?

   b. What factors allow you to come to this conclusion?

   c. What factors caused you to rule out other conditions?

d. What is the correct emergency treatment for this patient and in what order?

e. In what position will you transport this patient?

f. What continuing care will you provide for this patient en route to the hospital?

g. What common allied problems might you expect to find or see develop with this patient's condition?

h. What is the urgency of transportation to the hospital for this patient?

i. What would be your radio report to the hospital regarding the situation and present condition of the patient?

# 9

# Injuries II: Musculoskeletal Injuries The Upper Extremities

- The Musculoskeletal System
- Injuries to Bones and Joints
- Emergency Care for Injuries to the Extremities

---

1. Proper care of bone and joint injuries must:

    a. come before treatment of any other injuries.
    b. be always done with sterile materials.
    c. always involve straightening the limb to accomplish splinting.
    d. include efficient soft tissue care.

2. The anatomical term for the collarbone is:

    a. scapula.
    b. clavicle.
    c. carpal.
    d. sternum.

3. The number of bones in the human body is:

    a. 186.
    b. 200.
    c. 202.
    d. 206.

4. A sprain occurs when:

    a. ligaments are torn.
    b. muscles are torn.
    c. bones slide or are torn out of their joints.
    d. muscles are stretched.

5. The grating sound sometimes heard when a fractured limb is moved is:

    a. crepitus.
    b. synovial movement.
    c. not a sign of fracture.
    d. sign of a dislocation.

6. The EMT should care for a sprain:

    a. with an ace bandage.
    b. as a suspected fracture.
    c. with moist heat.
    d. by having the patient "work out" the pain.

7. When an EMT comes upon a patient with an obvious fracture, he should first:

    a. conduct a primary survey.
    b. check the pulse below the fracture.
    c. straighten the fracture.
    d. splint the fracture.

8. Swelling and the formation of a blood clot in the area of a fracture is due to loss of blood in adjacent blood vessels and:

    a. destruction of blood vessels in the periosteum.
    b. loss of fluid from the synovial joint.

c. destruction of blood vessels in the pericardium.
d. destruction of blood vessels in the phalanges.

9. A fracture where the bone ends have pushed through the skin and have been pulled back into the skin:
   a. is a closed fracture.
   b. is an open fracture.
   c. should not be covered with a sterile dressing to allow the EMT to view the fracture site.
   d. should be covered with a sterile dressing, but not splinted.

10. Which of the following injuries should the EMT attempt to straighten?
    a. Dislocations of the elbow if a radial pulse is not felt
    b. Angulated fractures of the wrist
    c. Dislocations of the shoulder
    d. Open fractures

11. The EMT has splinted a closed fracture of the humerus and finds that the radial pulse can no longer be felt. He or she should:
    a. transport immediately.
    b. resplint and check the pulse; if no pulse, transport immediately.
    c. continue to treat all other injuries.
    d. loosen the splint and transport.

12. Which of the following statements concerning fractures is true?
    a. Fractures can be different from dislocations easily.
    b. Few fractures present a real threat to life.
    c. All angulated fractures should be straightened.
    d. Fractures should be reduced by the EMT.

13. A major disadvantage of the airsplint when used in cold weather is that:
    a. once the patient is moved into the ambulance, the increased pressure may cut off circulation.
    b. once the patient is moved into the ambulance, the higher temperature will result in less firmness and support.
    c. the material will feel too cool for patient comfort.
    d. the material cracks.

14. The formation of a joint where two or more bones come together is called:
    a. articulation.
    b. appendicular.
    c. crepitus.
    d. angulation.

15. How many finger bones are there in each hand?
    a. 5
    b. 8
    c. 14
    d. 16

16. When splinting a fractured hand, the hand should:
    a. be splinted midway to the elbow.
    b. not be totally immobilized to allow movement for the fingers.
    c. be kept in the position of function.
    d. be covered only on the sides of the hand.

17. The anatomical term for the medial bone of the lower arm is the:
    a. radius.
    b. ulna.
    c. humerus.
    d. clavicle.

18. Black-and-blue discoloration associated with a fracture usually develops:
    a. immediately.
    b. within a few minutes.
    c. after several hours.
    d. after 24 hours.

19. The EMT should immobilize a fractured elbow:
    a. in the position it is found.
    b. in the position of function.
    c. with an airsplint.
    d. after it has been gently straightened.

20. Bone marrow is located in the long bones in a cavity called the:
    a. marrow cavity.
    b. articular canal.
    c. medullary canal.
    d. periosteum.

21. The treatment for a dislocated elbow is:
    a. reduce the dislocation, then transport.
    b. reduce the dislocation, splint, and then transport.
    c. splint the dislocation in the position it is found.
    d. let the patient hold the arm himself.

22. The EMT should inflate an airsplint until:
    a. wrinkles in the splint are ready to disappear.
    b. wrinkles in the splint have just disappeared.

## 58 INJURIES II: MUSCULOSKELETAL INJURIES

    c. the splint can be slightly dented with moderate thumb pressure.
    d. the splint is rigid and cannot be dented with thumb pressure.

23. The bones of the wrist are called:
    a. carpals.
    b. metacarpals.
    c. tarsals.
    d. metatarsals.

24. The primary reason that the EMT does not attempt to straighten a dislocation is that this may cause:
    a. severe pain.
    b. further nerve and blood vessel damage.
    c. severe bone damage.
    d. shock.

25. To immobilize a fractured clavicle the EMT should apply:
    a. a sling and swathe.
    b. an airsplint to the entire arm.
    c. a traction splint to the arm on the injured side.
    d. a sling.

26. The ends of bones forming joints are covered with:
    a. the periosteum.
    b. articular cartilage.
    c. smooth muscles.
    d. bone marrow.

27. A frozen or locked joint is usually a sign of:
    a. muscle spasms.
    b. fracture.
    c. dislocation.
    d. swelling.

28. The EMT should splint a colles fracture by:
    a. using an airsplint.
    b. using a traction splint.
    c. using a scoop-type stretcher.
    d. splinting it as he or she found it.

29. How many bones make up each ankle?
    a. 6
    b. 7
    c. 8
    d. 10

30. Bones are covered by a strong, white, fibrous material called:
    a. cartilage.
    b. ligaments.
    c. the periosteum.
    d. bone marrow.

31. In addition to checking skin color and nail bed color below the fracture site for signs of impaired circulation, the EMT should:
    a. palpate the pulse distal to the fracture.
    b. palpate the pulse proximal to the fracture.
    c. palpate the pulse on the uninjured side.
    d. not be concerned with impaired circulation, since immobilization of the fracture is much more important.

### SITUATIONS FOR FURTHER DISCUSSION

1. You are called to treat the victim of a fall. Your survey indicates an open fracture of the lower right arm. The wound does not appear to have hemorrhaged much. The radial pulse on the injured side is normal compared to the uninjured side's radial pulse. The patient also is suspected of having suffered a shoulder dislocation to the right shoulder.

    a. What do your primary and secondary surveys indicate the problem to be?

    b. What factors allow you to come to this conclusion?

    c. What factors caused you to rule out other conditions?

d. What is the correct emergency treatment for this patient and in what order?

e. In what position will you transport this patient?

f. What continuing care will you provide for this patient en route to the hospital?

g. What common allied problems might you expect to find or see develop with this patient's condition?

h. What is the urgency of transportation to the hospital for this patient?

i. What would be your radio report to the hospital regarding the situation and present condition of the patient?

# 10

# Injuries II: The Lower Extremities

- *The Lower Extremities*
- *Splinting the Lower Extremities*
- *Injuries of the Lower Extremities*

---

1. The EMT finds a patient with an anterior hip dislocation. In this situation:

   a. the leg is rotated inward.
   b. the leg is shortened and rotated inward.
   c. the entire lower limb is rotated outward.
   d. there is damage to the sciatic nerve.

2. A 70-year-old patient slips on a small rug and falls on her side. You notice that her left leg is slightly shorter than the right leg and is rotated outward. She most likely has suffered a:

   a. fractured pelvis.
   b. dislocated hip.
   c. fractured hip.
   d. fractured tibia and fibula.

3. Which of the following would have the highest priority of treatment?

   a. Fractures of the spine
   b. Fractures of a rib
   c. Fractures of the femur
   d. Multiple fractures of the extremities

4. The preferred treatment for a fracture of the femur is:

   a. full leg airsplint.
   b. cardboard splint.
   c. immobilization on a long board.
   d. traction splint.

5. If the EMT applies gentle traction to a fractured femur, the traction should be:

   a. loosened every 15 minutes.
   b. maintained at the same tension until arrival at the hospital.
   c. gradually tightened every 30 minutes.
   d. never maintained for more than one hour.

6. The EMT should apply mechanical traction to a closed femur fracture using a Hare traction splint until:

   a. the leg is noticeably stretched.
   b. the bone ends realign.
   c. the knurled knob no longer turns manually.
   d. manual traction is equalled and pain and muscle spasm are reduced.

7. The EMT should immobilize a fracture or dislocation of the knee by:

   a. lifting the patient with a scoop-type stretcher.
   b. splinting the fracture in the position found.
   c. using an airsplint.
   d. using sand bags.

8. The term used to describe the kneecap is:

   a. periosteum.
   b. patella.
   c. synovial joint.
   d. scapula.

## SITUATIONS FOR FURTHER DISCUSSION

1. You must treat the victim of a motorcycle accident who appears to have a fracture of the right femur (closed) and an open fracture to the right lower leg just above the ankle. The patient's vitals indicate near-shock levels.

   a. What do your primary and secondary surveys indicate the problem to be?

   b. What factors allow you to come to this conclusion?

   c. What factors caused you to rule out other conditions?

   d. What is the correct emergency treatment for this patient and in what order?

   e. In what position will you transport this patient?

   f. What continuing care will you provide for this patient en route to the hospital?

   g. What common allied problems might you expect to find or see develop with this patient's condition?

   h. What is the urgency of transportation to the hospital for this patient?

   i. What would be your radio report to the hospital regarding the situation and present condition of the patient?

2. You are called to the home of an elderly woman by family members who haven't been able to reach her by phone for the past day. When you arrive, you find the woman lying on the floor on her side and in a great deal of pain. She is conscious and alert but unable to move. Her left leg appears shortened and externally rotated. No other injuries can be found.

   a. What do your primary and secondary surveys indicate the problem to be?

   b. What factors allow you to come to this conclusion?

   c. What factors caused you to rule out other conditions?

## 62 INJURIES II: THE LOWER EXTREMITIES

d. What is the correct emergency treatment for this patient and in what order?

e. In what position will you transport this patient?

f. What continuing care will you provide for this patient en route to the hospital?

g. What common allied problems might you expect to find or see develop with this patient's condition?

h. What is the urgency of transportation to the hospital for this patient?

i. What would be your radio report to the hospital regarding the situation and present condition of the patient?

# 11

# Injuries III: The Skull and Spine

- Axial Skeleton
- The Nervous System
- Injuries to the Skull and Brain
- Care for Head Injuries
- Injuries to the Spine
- Care for Spinal Injuries

---

1. The skull, spinal column, ribs, and sternum make up the:

    a. appendicular skeleton.
    b. axial skeleton.
    c. vertebral column.
    d. thoracic cavity.

2. The skull is made up of:

    a. 12 bones.
    b. 20 bones.
    c. 22 bones.
    d. 24 bones.

3. The bony extensions of the posterior vertebrae are called:

    a. fontanels.
    b. sphenoid fontanels.
    c. costal arches.
    d. spinous processes.

4. The central nervous system is comprised of the:

    a. brain only.
    b. brain and spinal cord.
    c. brain, spinal cord, and optic nerve.
    d. spinal cord only.

5. A brain contusion usually develops on the side:

    a. opposite from impact and is a closed head injury.
    b. opposite from impact and is an open head injury.
    c. near to impact and is a closed head injury.
    d. near to impact and is an open head injury.

6. The point at which two bones of the cranium articulate is called:

    a. suture.
    b. meninges.
    c. orbit.
    d. fusion.

7. The spinal column is comprised of:

    a. two regions.
    b. three regions.
    c. four regions.
    d. five regions.

8. Fractures to the cranium floor are called:

    a. linear skull fractures.
    b. comminuted skull fractures.
    c. basal skull fractures.
    d. facial skull fractures.

## 64 INJURIES III: THE SKULL AND SPINE

9. Clear fluid flowing from the ears of a head-injured patient is probably:

    a. plasma.
    b. cerebrospinal fluid.
    c. water.
    d. not related to the head injury.

10. A subdural hematoma occurs when blood from damaged blood vessels and tissues collects between the:

    a. scalp and cranial bones.
    b. brain and meninges.
    c. meninges and the cranial bones.
    d. brain tissues.

11. The EMT must assume that any unconscious patient who is the victim of an accident:

    a. is in shock.
    b. has to be transported immediately.
    c. has spinal injuries.
    d. should be kept in a seated position.

12. Which of the following is a sign of brain injury?

    a. Personality changes
    b. Low blood pressure
    c. Lowered body temperature
    d. Heart rate becomes slow and weak

13. An epidural hematoma occurs when the blood flows between the:

    a. meninges and the cranial bones.
    b. meninges and the brain.
    c. scalp and the cranial bones.
    d. brain tissues.

14. The lumbar region of the spine contains:

    a. four vertebrae.
    b. five vertebrae.
    c. six vertebrae.
    d. seven vertebrae.

15. A skull fracture with cracks radiating out from the center of the point of impact is called a:

    a. linear skull fracture.
    b. comminuted skull fracture.
    c. depressed skull fracture.
    d. basal skull fracture.

16. During the survey of the skull, the EMT detects severe pain and swelling. He or she should:

    a. not palpate the injury site.
    b. palpate the area to detect the cause of pain.
    c. palpate the area thoroughly to detect impaled objects such as glass.
    d. apply direct pressure to reduce the swelling.

17. The spinal column is made up of:

    a. 16 bones.
    b. 24 bones.
    c. 33 bones.
    d. 42 bones.

18. For all patients with possible spinal injuries, the EMT should:

    a. administer oxygen in high concentrations.
    b. apply a cervical collar and release manual traction.
    c. hyperextend the neck to assure an open airway.
    d. allow the patient to walk with assistance to the ambulance if the patient can feel and move his/her extremities.

19. To determine the proper size extrication collar, the EMT should be sure the collar:

    a. fits from the chin to the jugular notch.
    b. fits from the trachea to the sternum.
    c. completely covers the ears.
    d. is loose enough so the carotid pulse can be checked.

20. The EMT tests for response to painful stimuli at the bottom of each foot. If there is reaction to the stimuli by slight pulling back of the foot, it may indicate that:

    a. the spinal cord is severed.
    b. the spinal cord is intact at present.
    c. the patient may be moved without spinal immobilization.
    d. the spinal column is not injured.

21. The spinal column contains:

    a. 8 cervical vertebrae.
    b. 12 thoracic vertebrae.
    c. 4 lumbar vertebrae.
    d. 13 thoracic vertebrae.

22. Which parts of the spine are more susceptible to injury?

    a. Cervical and thoracic
    b. Cervical and lumbar
    c. Thoracic and lumbar
    d. Thoracic and sacral

## SITUATIONS FOR FURTHER DISCUSSION

1. The victim of a motorcycle accident is found with loss of sensation in both lower extremities. He is found lying on his back with no other obvious injury. He is still wearing a helmet.

   a. What do your primary and secondary surveys indicate the problem to be?

   b. What factors allow you to come to this conclusion?

   c. What factors caused you to rule out other conditions?

   d. What is the correct emergency treatment for this patient and in what order?

   e. In what position will you transport this patient?

   f. What continuing care will you provide for this patient en route to the hospital?

   g. What common allied problems might you expect to find or see develop with this patient's condition?

   h. What is the urgency of transportation to the hospital for this patient?

   i. What would be your radio report to the hospital regarding the situation and present condition of the patient?

2. A 24-year-old male from a snowmobile accident is found to have trouble breathing, severe neck pain, and possible signs of cervical spine injury. Witnesses state that the patient ran into a rope stretched across the trail that hit him in the neck. The patient appears slightly cyanotic.

   a. What do your primary and secondary surveys indicate the problem to be?

   b. What factors allow you to come to this conclusion?

   c. What factors caused you to rule out other conditions?

## 66 INJURIES III: THE SKULL AND SPINE

d. What is the correct emergency treatment for this patient and in what order?

e. In what position will you transport this patient?

f. What continuing care will you provide for this patient en route to the hospital?

g. What common allied problems might you expect to find or see develop with this patient's condition?

h. What is the urgency of transportation to the hospital for this patient?

i. What would be your radio report to the hospital regarding the situation and present condition of the patient?

# 12

# Injuries III: Soft Tissue Injuries of the Head and Neck

- *Injuries to the Soft Tissues of the Head*
- *Injuries to the Soft Tissues of the Neck*

---

1. When treating a patient with a head wound and possible spinal injury, the EMT should:
   a. lift the head steadily to access and clean a scalp wound.
   b. wrap the patient's scalp wound using a snug pressure dressing to control bleeding.
   c. not lift or attempt to wrap the patient's head.
   d. move the unconscious patient with head trauma into a head-raised position.

2. The auricle is also referred to as the:
   a. pinna.
   b. patella.
   c. oviduct.
   d. eardrum.

3. In situations where the patient's tooth is avulsed:
   a. wrap the tooth in dry dressings and transport with the patient.
   b. wrap the tooth in moist dressings and transport with the patient.
   c. rub the tooth in attempts to clean it.
   d. insert cotton packets into the socket to control bleeding.

4. The white portion of the eye is called the:
   a. cornea.
   b. sclera.
   c. pupil.
   d. iris.

5. When treating a patient with an avulsed eye, the EMT should:
   a. try to replace the eye in its socket.
   b. cover the avulsed eye with a snug, sterile dressing to keep it in place.
   c. treat the avulsed eye in the same manner as you would treat an impaled object in the eye.
   d. close both eyelids and cover both eyes with sterile dressings taped in place.

6. Clear or bloody fluids coming from the ear must be considered by the EMT to be a sign of:
   a. skull fracture.
   b. ruptured tympanic membrane.
   c. middle ear infection.
   d. external acoustic meatus damage.

7. When the EMT is caring for a patient with chemical burns to the eye, the EMT should:
   a. flush the eyes with a steady stream of water for at least 20 minutes during transport.
   b. flush from the lateral to the medial corner of the eye.
   c. flush with a mild acidic solution if the burn was caused by a base.
   d. cover both eyes immediately to allow tearing to cleanse the eyes.

## 68   INJURIES III: SOFT TISSUE INJURIES OF THE HEAD AND NECK

8. The proper procedure to be followed by an EMT when caring for a patient who is bleeding from the ears is to:

   a. apply loose dressings to the external ear and bandage in place.
   b. irrigate the external ear canal using sterile water and a bulb syringe.
   c. pack the external ear canal with sterile gauze to stop the flow of blood.
   d. probe carefully to determine the source of hemorrhage.

9. Which of the following is the correct treatment for soft tissue injuries to the face?

   a. Always clear or clean the surface of a scalp wound.
   b. Apply finger pressure to a scalp wound to control bleeding.
   c. Remove objects impaled in the cheek if they enter the oral cavity.
   d. Control bleeding with sterile dressings held in place with tight pressure.

10. Severe trauma to the face may also produce:

    a. referred pain in the abdomen.
    b. airway obstruction.
    c. damage to the sciatic nerve.
    d. vomiting.

11. The colored portion of the anterior eye that adjusts the size of the pupil is the:

    a. cornea.
    b. sclera.
    c. iris.
    d. conjunctiva.

12. Care for nasal injuries is usually directed toward:

    a. maintaining an open airway.
    b. packing the nose with gauze.
    c. positioning the patient with the head tilted back.
    d. removal of protruding foreign objects.

13. The semirigid capsule of fibrous tissue that helps to maintain the shape of the globe of the eye and contains the fluids found inside the eye is the:

    a. sclera.
    b. cornea.
    c. conjunctiva.
    d. retina.

14. In situations where a patient is suffering from possible burns to the eyes caused by heat, the EMT must:

    a. flush the eyes with sterile water for at least 5 minutes.
    b. inspect the eyes if the eyelids are burned to determine the extent of damage.
    c. close the eyelids and apply loose, moist dressings to both eyes.
    d. cover both eyes with dry, sterile dressings.

15. The transparent covering over the iris and pupil of the eye is the:

    a. cornea.
    b. sclera.
    c. patella.
    d. retina.

16. When caring for a patient with light burns to the eyes, caused by an arc welder, the EMT should:

    a. cover the eyes with a loose, moist dressing.
    b. irrigate the eyes for at least 15 minutes, both at the scene and during transport.
    c. close the eyelids and apply dark patches over both eyes.
    d. put dark sunglasses on the patient.

17. The proper position for a patient suffering epistaxis, who also does not exhibit any signs or symptoms of skull fracture, is:

    a. seated with the head tilted back.
    b. seated, leaning slightly forward.
    c. lying in a supine position with the head erect.
    d. lying in the supine position, with the head tilted back.

18. When the EMT places gauze into a patient's mouth to control bleeding, it is important to remember that:

    a. objects such as gauze may become airway obstructions.
    b. only occlusive materials should be used.
    c. dressings must be held in place even if a gag reflex develops.
    d. a gastric tube should be in place.

19. A patient suffering epistaxis has:

    a. fainted.
    b. a nosebleed.
    c. a displaced kneecap.
    d. a hernia.

20. When removing flexible contact lenses, the EMT should remember that:
    a. a special suction cup is available for the removal of flexible contact lenses.
    b. flexible contact lenses must always be removed in any emergency.
    c. slide the flexible lens into the proper position for removal, directly over the cornea.
    d. compress the flexible lens slightly between the thumb and index finger, using a pinching motion.

21. If a foreign object protrudes from a patient's nostril, the EMT should:
    a. remove the object.
    b. probe to determine if the object has penetrated the septum, or tissues high in the nose.
    c. encourage the patient to forcefully blow his nose in an effort to dislodge the object.
    d. transport the patient without disturbing the object.

22. When irritated, the tiny blood vessels of the eye become swollen with blood, giving a "bloodshot" or pink appearance called:
    a. vitreous humor.
    b. conjunctivitis.
    c. membrane tympanica.
    d. retinal hemorrhage.

23. To control bleeding from the socket of a dislodged tooth for a conscious patient the EMT should:
    a. insert cotton packs into the socket.
    b. pinch the socket closed using the finger tips and a sterile dressing.
    c. have the patient bite down on a pad of sterile gauze placed over the socket.
    d. do not attempt to control the bleeding, since any attempt may disrupt the pocket tissues.

24. Which of the following is the proper procedure for removal of an object on the cornea?
    a. Use a sterile, moist applicator or gauze to carefully remove the foreign body.
    b. Probe carefully using a sterile cotton swab.
    c. Attempt to grasp the object using a sterile dressing.
    d. Do not attempt to remove an object on the cornea.

25. The EMT should consider a lacerated sclera to be a serious situation since a deep cut may:
    a. allow vitreous humor to escape.
    b. cause sympathetic eye movement.
    c. have also caused minor scratches to the surface of the eye.
    d. create pressure on the optic nerve.

26. To control a nosebleed, the EMT should:
    a. pack the nostrils.
    b. pinch the nostrils shut.
    c. do nothing, since this is usually self-correcting.
    d. place the patient in a supine position.

27. Subcutaneous emphysema is the result of:
    a. improper administration of oxygen, using a bag mask, demand valve, or other form of positive pressure resuscitation equipment.
    b. air leaking into the tissues of the neck.
    c. blood and fluids seeping into the tissues of the neck.
    d. a fractured skull.

28. When caring for a patient with facial wounds, if blood vessels, nerves, tendons, or muscles have been exposed, the EMT should:
    a. apply an ice pack.
    b. apply a sterile dressing moistened with sterile water.
    c. apply a sterile dressing moistened with sterile saline solution.
    d. apply a sterile dressing, then tin foil or plastic wrap over it, and seal the edges with tape.

29. When caring for eye injuries, the EMT must:
    a. cover both eyes, even if only one eye is injured.
    b. cover only the injured eye.
    c. obtain the hospital's permission prior to covering the eye.
    d. not cover the eyes.

30. If there are clear fluids coming from the nose or ears, or a mix of blood and clear fluids draining from the nose and ears, the proper procedure for the EMT to follow is:
    a. pack the nose to stop the flow.
    b. pinch the nostrils shut to control bleeding.
    c. do not attempt to stop the flow in any way.
    d. pack the external acoustic meatus to stop the escape of fluids.

31. Loss of the jelly-like vitreous humor due to an open wound of the eye can result in:
    a. conjunctivitis.
    b. blindness.
    c. sympathetic eye movement.
    d. an extended length of time before the body can produce more.

## 70 INJURIES III: SOFT TISSUE INJURIES OF THE HEAD AND NECK

32. When caring for patients with soft tissue injuries to the mouth who have problems involving teeth and dental appliances, the EMT should:
    a. search for and remove any dislodged teeth, crowns, and bridges.
    b. place cotton packets into tooth sockets to stop bleeding.
    c. rub dislodged teeth in sterile gauze to clean debris from the teeth.
    d. leave all dental appliances in the mouth since they may be aspirated during removal.

33. The emergency care for the eyes of an unconscious patient whose eyes are found open is to:
    a. irrigate the eyes with sterile water.
    b. irrigate the eyes with sterile saline solution.
    c. provide no care as long as the eyes are not injured.
    d. close the eyelids and keep them closed.

34. The emergency care to control bleeding from a severed neck artery includes application of:
    a. direct pressure and carotid artery pressure point techniques.
    b. direct pressure over the trachea.
    c. direct pressure over both sides of the neck simultaneously.
    d. facial artery pressure point techniques.

35. The proper position for hard contact lenses as they are being removed is:
    a. on the sclera.
    b. directly over the cornea.
    c. partially covering the cornea and sclera.
    d. There is not a special position.

36. To control bleeding from a neck vein the EMT must:
    a. apply direct pressure on the carotid arteries on both sides of the neck.
    b. apply a snug pressure dressing around the neck.
    c. apply an occlusive dressing or plastic wrap over the injury site and tape the dressing on all sides so it is airtight.
    d. transport immediately and administer high concentrations of oxygen, since there is no effective way to control bleeding from a neck vein.

37. Injury to the eye may mean that:
    a. the injured eye may have to be kept open.
    b. small amounts of lost aqueous humor cannot be replaced.
    c. there may also be injuries to the cervical spine.
    d. impaled objects should be removed and both eyes covered.

38. When caring for patients with injuries to the cranium, the EMT should:
    a. also treat neck and spinal injuries.
    b. stop the flow of all fluids from the ears.
    c. remove any impaled objects.
    d. apply direct pressure to control all scalp bleeding.

39. The major concern when the EMT deals with a patient who has suffered a facial fracture is:
    a. loss of sight.
    b. state of the airway.
    c. contamination.
    d. swelling.

40. The EMT may remove objects impaled in the:
    a. skull with profuse bleeding.
    b. face.
    c. soft tissues of the cheek.
    d. chest.

41. An unconscious patient with facial injuries and suspected spine injuries should be transported in the traumatic coma position:
    a. with the injured side of the face down.
    b. with the uninjured side of the face down.
    c. on a spineboard.
    d. without a cervical collar.

### SITUATIONS FOR FURTHER DISCUSSION

1. A 15-year-old boy has a sliver of glass impaled in his cheek. When you first arrive his breathing is noisy with gurgling sounds. His vitals are normal except for a rapid yet strong pulse.

   a. What do your primary and secondary surveys indicate the problem to be?

   b. What factors allow you to come to this conclusion?

## INJURIES III: SOFT TISSUE INJURIES OF THE HEAD AND NECK 71

c. What factors caused you to rule out other conditions?

d. What is the correct emergency treatment for this patient and in what order?

e. In what position will you transport this patient?

f. What continuing care will you provide for this patient en route to the hospital?

g. What common allied problems might you expect to find or see develop with this patient's condition?

h. What is the urgency of transportation to the hospital for this patient?

i. What would be your radio report to the hospital regarding the situation and present condition of the patient?

2. A 35-year-old woman in an automobile accident is found to have an object impaled in her left eye. She appears conscious, alert, and remarkably calm. Her vitals indicate a rapid, weak pulse and no signs of cyanosis. No other injuries are found.

   a. What do your primary and secondary surveys indicate the problem to be?

   b. What factors allow you to come to this conclusion?

   c. What factors caused you to rule out other conditions?

   d. What is the correct emergency treatment for this patient and in what order?

   e. In what position will you transport this patient?

   f. What continuing care will you provide for this patient en route to the hospital?

## 72  INJURIES III: SOFT TISSUE INJURIES OF THE HEAD AND NECK

g. What common allied problems might you expect to find or see develop with this patient's condition?

h. What is the urgency of transportation to the hospital for this patient?

i. What would be your radio report to the hospital regarding the situation and present condition of the patient?

3. While treating an unconscious patient, your partner finds that the patient is wearing contact lenses. No injuries are found in this patient and it is suspected that he has suffered from a medical problem.

   a. What do your primary and secondary surveys indicate the problem to be?

   b. What factors allow you to come to this conclusion?

   c. What factors caused you to rule out other conditions?

d. What is the correct emergency treatment for this patient and in what order?

e. In what position will you transport this patient?

f. What continuing care will you provide for this patient en route to the hospital?

g. What common allied problems might you expect to find or see develop with this patient's condition?

h. What is the urgency of transportation to the hospital for this patient?

i. What would be your radio report to the hospital regarding the situation and present condition of the patient?

INJURIES III: SOFT TISSUE INJURIES OF THE HEAD AND NECK  73

4. A patient is found who has severe epistaxis and no signs of head or neck injury.

   a. What do your primary and secondary surveys indicate the problem to be?

   b. What factors allow you to come to this conclusion?

   c. What factors caused you to rule out other conditions?

   d. What is the correct emergency treatment for this patient and in what order?

   e. In what position will you transport this patient?

   f. What continuing care will you provide for this patient en route to the hospital?

   g. What common allied problems might you expect to find or see develop with this patient's condition?

   h. What is the urgency of transportation to the hospital for this patient?

   i. What would be your radio report to the hospital regarding the situation and present condition of the patient?

5. You are called to treat the victim of a knifing. The patient is found in a large pool of blood and is unconscious. Your survey indicates that the neck is lacerated and that bleeding is coming from the major artery and vein in the neck. No other injuries are found.

   a. What do your primary and secondary surveys indicate the problem to be?

   b. What factors allow you to come to this conclusion?

   c. What factors caused you to rule out other conditions?

   d. What is the correct emergency treatment for this patient and in what order?

**74** INJURIES III: SOFT TISSUE INJURIES OF THE HEAD AND NECK

e. In what position will you transport this patient?

f. What continuing care will you provide for this patient en route to the hospital?

g. What common allied problems might you expect to find or see develop with this patient's condition?

h. What is the urgency of transportation to the hospital for this patient?

i. What would be your radio report to the hospital regarding the situation and present condition of the patient?

6. A 20-year-old male is seen who has been struck in the mouth with a bat during a baseball game. The patient is conscious, with obvious deformity to the lower jaw. Pulse and blood pressure appear normal, but respirations are noisy and irregular.

   a. What do your primary and secondary surveys indicate the problem to be?

b. What factors allow you to come to this conclusion?

c. What factors caused you to rule out other conditions?

d. What is the correct emergency treatment for this patient and in what order?

e. In what position will you transport this patient?

f. What continuing care will you provide for this patient en route to the hospital?

g. What common allied problems might you expect to find or see develop with this patient's condition?

h. What is the urgency of transportation to the hospital for this patient?

# INJURIES III: SOFT TISSUE INJURIES OF THE HEAD AND NECK

i. What would be your radio report to the hospital regarding the situation and present condition of the patient?

7. An unconscious victim is found who exhibits discoloration of the soft tissue under the eyes. Vitals appear normal and no other injuries are detected by your survey.

   a. What do your primary and secondary surveys indicate the problem to be?

   b. What factors allow you to come to this conclusion?

   c. What factors caused you to rule out other conditions?

   d. What is the correct emergency treatment for this patient and in what order?

   e. In what position will you transport this patient?

   f. What continuing care will you provide for this patient en route to the hospital?

   g. What common allied problems might you expect to find or see develop with this patient's condition?

   h. What is the urgency of transportation to the hospital for this patient?

   i. What would be your radio report to the hospital regarding the situation and present condition of the patient?

# 13

# Injuries IV: The Chest, Abdomen, and Genitalia

- *Injuries to the Chest*
- *Injuries to the Abdomen*
- *Injuries to the Pelvis and Groin*

---

1. A pear-shaped abdominal organ that is a reservoir for bile, located on the posterior undersurface of the liver is the:

   a. stomach.
   b. small intestine.
   c. gallbladder.
   d. duodenum.

2. The large, multifunctional, extremely vascular gland located in the right upper abdominal quadrant is the:

   a. liver.
   b. spleen.
   c. pancreas.
   d. gallbladder.

3. The emergency care for closed abdominal injuries includes:

   a. placing the patient on his back with the legs flexed at the knees, keeping alert for vomiting.
   b. treating for shock, administering small sips of water, monitoring vitals.
   c. applying a bulky pad snugly in place with tape, lying the patient in a prone position with the legs flexed.
   d. placing the patient on the injured side, administering salted water, monitoring vitals, and treating for shock.

4. The EMT should consider back pain following blunt trauma to be an indication of possible:

   a. kidney damage.
   b. abdominal injuries.
   c. referred pain.
   d. pelvic damage.

5. The elongated, flat, triangular gland, involved in producing insulin that lies in the abdominal cavity behind the stomach is the:

   a. spleen.
   b. liver.
   c. pancreas.
   d. appendix.

6. Which type of wound occurs when the intestine or other internal organ protrudes through an incision or wound in the abdomen?

   a. Inguinal hernia
   b. Evisceration
   c. Contusion
   d. Abrasion

7. The EMT should treat open abdominal wounds by:

   a. controlling external bleeding and dressing all open wounds.
   b. removing any impaled object in the abdomen so the wound may be covered with a sterile dressing.

c. lying the patient in a prone position.
d. placing any organs found outside the wound back into the abdomen.

8. A soft tissue injury in which the lining of the abdominopelvic cavity rupture and the intestine protrudes through the opening is called an:
   a. inguinal hernia.
   b. evisceration.
   c. avulsion.
   d. appendicitis injury.

9. The signs and symptoms of abdominal injury can include:
   a. obvious lacerations and puncture wounds to the abdomen; deep, gasping, labored breathing.
   b. rigid and/or tender abdomen, low blood pressure, coughing up blood.
   c. guarded abdomen; slow, full pulse; patient tries to be active.
   d. low blood pressure, rales, and cyanosis.

10. The injury which occurs when the pleural sac is punctured and air enters the thoracic cavity is called:
    a. a flail chest.
    b. dyspnea.
    c. a hemothorax.
    d. a pneumothorax.

11. Patients suffering from a flail chest often exhibit a section of the chest wall which moves in the opposite direction to the rest of the chest wall. This condition is:
    a. normal for this injury and is not serious.
    b. called paradoxical respiration.
    c. only serious if there is also an open chest wound.
    d. called a hemopneumothorax.

12. The EMT notices that the trachea appears to be pushed to one side in a patient who also has suffered chest trauma. This may indicate:
    a. dyspnea.
    b. a hemothorax.
    c. a tension pneumothorax.
    d. The patient probably was hit in the throat.

13. If the EMT finds that successive blood pressure measurements indicate systolic and diastolic readings that approach each other as the patient's condition deteriorates, he or she should suspect a:
    a. hemothorax.
    b. flail chest.
    c. cardiac tamponade.
    d. pneumothorax.

14. When three or more consecutive ribs on the same side of the chest are fractured, each in at least two places, the injury is called:
    a. a pneumothorax.
    b. a paradoxical chest.
    c. a traumatic asphyxia.
    d. a flail chest.

15. If the patient deteriorates rapidly after the EMT seals a sucking chest wound with an occlusive dressing, the EMT should:
    a. rush the patient to the hospital.
    b. administer positive pressure oxygen.
    c. quickly unseal the occlusive dressing and reseal the wound when the tension improves.
    d. remove the occlusive dressing and rush the patient to the hospital.

16. The EMT should consider it critical if a patient's pulse pressure is below:
    a. 90 mmHg.
    b. 60 mmHg.
    c. 30 mmHg.
    d. 15 mmHg.

17. When the EMT treats a patient suffering a pneumothorax, the last edge of the occlusive dressing should be:
    a. left unsealed.
    b. sealed with tape when the patient forcefully exhales.
    c. sealed with tape when the patient inhales.
    d. sealed with tape only if the blood pressure is below 90 mmHg systolic.

18. An impaled object found in the chest should be:
    a. removed so an occlusive dressing can be applied.
    b. placed flat against the chest and secured to reduce movement.
    c. left in place and supported with bulky dressings and securely held in place using tape or cravates.
    d. cut off at the skin to reduce movement and to allow for a complete seal with an occlusive dressing.

19. The ribs that are most commonly fractured are the:
    a. upper four pairs.
    b. fifth through tenth pairs.
    c. first and second pairs.
    d. floating ribs.

# 78 INJURIES IV: THE CHEST, ABDOMEN, AND GENITALIA

20. The term floating ribs is given to:
    a. the lower two pairs of ribs.
    b. the lower three pairs of ribs.
    c. the lower four pairs of ribs.
    d. the lower pair of ribs.

21. To treat suspected fractured ribs, the EMT secures the:
    a. arm on the injured side to the chest with three cravates.
    b. arm on the uninjured side to the chest with three cravates.
    c. ribs with a single wide cravate.
    d. arm on the uninjured side to the chest with four cravates.

## SITUATIONS FOR FURTHER DISCUSSION

1. The victim of a gunshot wound to the chest exhibits a sucking sound from both the front and back of his chest.

    a. What do your primary and secondary surveys indicate the problem to be?

    b. What factors allow you to come to this conclusion?

    c. What factors caused you to rule out other conditions?

    d. What is the correct emergency treatment for this patient and in what order?

    e. In what position will you transport this patient?

    f. What continuing care will you provide for this patient en route to the hospital?

    g. What common allied problems might you expect to find or see develop with this patient's condition?

    h. What is the urgency of transportation to the hospital for this patient?

    i. What would be your radio report to the hospital regarding the situation and present condition of the patient?

2. The driver of a car involved in a head-on collision is found to be cyanotic and unconscious. A segment of his chest bulges when he exhales and depresses when he inhales.

    a. What do your primary and secondary surveys indicate the problem to be?

## INJURIES IV: THE CHEST, ABDOMEN, AND GENITALIA 79

b. What factors allow you to come to this conclusion?

c. What factors caused you to rule out other conditions?

d. What is the correct emergency treatment for this patient and in what order?

e. In what position will you transport this patient?

f. What continuing care will you provide for this patient en route to the hospital?

g. What common allied problems might you expect to find or see develop with this patient's condition?

h. What is the urgency of transportation to the hospital for this patient?

i. What would be your radio report to the hospital regarding the situation and present condition of the patient?

3. While treating the patient in situation #2, it is noted that the initial blood pressure was 100/60 mmHg. Now, five minutes later, the blood pressure is 90/80 mmHg.

   a. What do your primary and secondary surveys indicate the problem to be?

   b. What factors allow you to come to this conclusion?

   c. What factors caused you to rule out other conditions?

   d. What is the correct emergency treatment for this patient and in what order?

   e. In what position will you transport this patient?

## 80 INURIES IV: THE CHEST, ABDOMEN, AND GENITALIA

f. What continuing care will you provide for this patient en route to the hospital?

g. What common allied problems might you expect to find or see develop with this patient's condition?

h. What is the urgency of transportation to the hospital for this patient?

i. What would be your radio report to the hospital regarding the situation and present condition of the patient?

# 14

# Medical Emergencies

## SECTION ONE: MEDICAL EMERGENCIES

- *What Are Medical Emergencies?*
- *Poisoning*
- *Disorders of the Cardiovascular System*
- *Respiratory System Disorders*

---

1. The condition that may be due to the long-term reactions of tissues in the respiratory tract to smoking, allergens, chemical, air pollutants, or repeated infections is:

    a. chronic obstructive pulmonary disease.
    b. asthma.
    c. dyspnea.
    d. respiratory insufficiency.

2. "Hardening of the arteries" caused by calcium deposits is called:

    a. atherosclerosis.
    b. arteriosclerosis.
    c. chronic bronchitis.
    d. emphysema.

3. In which medical emergency does the pain generally diminish and disappear when physical or emotional stress ends and seldom lasts no more than 3 to 5 minutes?

    a. Chronic emphysema
    b. Congestive heart failure
    c. Angina pectoris
    d. Acute myocardial infarction

4. The EMT must assume there is a medical emergency and transport the patient to the hospital for definitive care when the patient:

    a. refuses your care.
    b. has typical vital signs.
    c. says that he or she is not feeling "normal" in any way.
    d. is under the care of a physician.

5. An arrhythmia that occurs when the ventricles no longer beat with a full, steady, symmetrical pattern is:

    a. bradycardia.
    b. tachycardia.
    c. atrial fibrillation.
    d. ventricular fibrillation.

6. The sharp chest pain occurring when a portion of the myocardium is not receiving enough oxygenated blood is:

    a. rales.
    b. dyspnea.
    c. ascites.
    d. angina pectoris.

## 82 MEDICAL EMERGENCIES SECTION ONE

7. Medical problems present over a long period of time are:
   a. acute.
   b. congenital.
   c. chronic.
   d. episodic.

8. One type of cardiovascular system disorder stems from weakened sections in the arterial walls. Each weak spot that begins to dilate is called:
   a. an embolus.
   b. a thrombus.
   c. an angina.
   d. an aneurysm.

9. The condition in which a portion of the myocardium dies when deprived of oxygenated blood is:
   a. arteriosclerosis.
   b. atherosclerosis.
   c. acute myocardial infarction.
   d. asystole.

10. Medical problems affecting the patient at irregular intervals yet leaving him unaffected at other times are:
    a. acute.
    b. chronic.
    c. congenital.
    d. episodic.

11. A major factor in heart disease is sudden death or cardiac arrest that occurs within:
    a. 5 minutes of the onset of symptoms.
    b. 1 hour of the onset of symptoms.
    c. 2 hours of the onset of symptoms.
    d. 4 hours of the onset of symptoms.

12. The failure of the heart to pump efficiently, leading to excessive blood or fluid in the lungs and/or the body is called:
    a. chronic obstructive pulmonary disease.
    b. cerebrovascular accident.
    c. congestive heart failure.
    d. pericardial tamponade.

13. If a known coronary bypass patient suffers a cardiac arrest, the EMT should:
    a. not perform CPR due to the risk of further injury.
    b. deliver light compressions due to the risk of further injury.
    c. provide CPR in the same manner as you would do for any other arrested patient.
    d. provide CPR unless the fracture of the sternum or ribs becomes apparent.

14. A hyperventilating patient breathes too:
    a. rapidly and deeply.
    b. rapidly and shallowly.
    c. slowly and shallowly.
    d. slowly and deeply.

15. The term used to describe labored or difficult breathing is:
    a. apnea.
    b. dyspnea.
    c. asphyxia.
    d. rales.

16. Blood clots and debris from plaque in a diseased artery can form an obstruction that can reach a size where it occludes blood flow completely. This occlusion is called a(n):
    a. arrhythmia.
    b. embolus.
    c. thrombus.
    d. aneurysm.

17. A patient suffering from congestive heart failure may exhibit abnormal breathing sounds which sound powdery or gravelly when auscultated with a stethoscope. These sounds are called:
    a. edema.
    b. rales.
    c. ascites.
    d. snoring.

18. Asystole means:
    a. difficult, labored breathing.
    b. the abdomen becomes noticeably distended by fluids.
    c. the patient is hyperventilating.
    d. cardiac standstill.

19. A heart rate below 40 or 50 beats per minutes is called:
    a. bradycardia.
    b. tachycardia.
    c. asystole.
    d. ventricular fibrillation.

20. When providing emergency care and transportation to the stroke patient, the EMT should:
    a. calm and reassure them.
    b. transport rapidly.

c. transport rapidly, with sirens.
d. apply rotating tourniquets.

21. The proper emergency medical care for a patient who is hyperventilating is:

    a. administer 24 percent oxygen by venturi mask.
    b. administer 100 percent oxygen.
    c. have the patient breathe into a paper bag.
    d. administer nitroglycerine under the patient's tongue.

22. Medical problems occurring suddenly, without warning, are:

    a. acute.
    b. chronic.
    c. episodic.
    d. congenital.

23. When a thrombus breaks loose from a diseased artery and moves to occlude the flow of blood in a smaller artery, it is called an:

    a. aneurysm.
    b. asystole.
    c. embolus.
    d. arrhythmia.

24. The buildup of fatty deposits and other particles (plaque) on the inner wall of the artery is known as:

    a. atherosclerosis.
    b. arteriosclerosis.
    c. edema.
    d. ascites.

25. A patient experiencing headache, confusion, loss of function on one side, loss of facial expression, impaired speech, unequal pupils, rapid pulse, and difficult respirations is suffering:

    a. right heart failure.
    b. alcohol intoxication.
    c. spinal injury.
    d. cerebrovascular accident.

26. Which disease may be triggered by an allergic reaction to something inhaled, swallowed, or injected into the body?

    a. Emphysema
    b. Angina pectoris
    c. Asthma
    d. Chronic bronchitis

27. What medication is prescribed to dilate the coronary arteries in patients who suffer angina attacks?

    a. Aspirin
    b. Nitroglycerin
    c. Oxygen
    d. Valium

28. A defect in the structure or function of an organ or organ system that is present at birth is:

    a. acute.
    b. chronic.
    c. episodic.
    d. congenital.

29. A heart rate exceeding 120 beats per minute is called:

    a. bradycardia.
    b. tachycardia.
    c. asystole.
    d. atrial fibrillation.

30. Which medical emergency is the result of damage to one of the arteries supplying oxygenated blood to the brain?

    a. Apnea
    b. Asthma
    c. Cerebrovascular accident
    d. Diabetes mellitus

31. The medical emergency often associated with cardiac arrhythmias, and pain that may occur even when the patient is at rest, is called:

    a. angina pectoris.
    b. congestive heart failure.
    c. acute myocardial infarction.
    d. emphysema.

32. Temporary cessation of breathing is called:

    a. apnea.
    b. dyspnea.
    c. rales.
    d. pulmonary edema.

33. The signs and symptoms of congestive heart failure can include:

    a. dyspnea, pulmonary edema with rales, occasional coughing up pink sputum.
    b. anxiety or confusion, bradycardia, edema of the lower extremities.
    c. cyanosis, low blood pressure, enlarged liver and spleen, abdominal distention.
    d. edema of lower extremities, cyanosis, anxiety, deep respirations, bradycardia.

## 84 MEDICAL EMERGENCIES SECTION ONE

34. What special care is necessary for patients with the signs and symptoms of acute myocardial infarction, angina pectoris, or chronic heart failure, if the patient wears a cardiac pacemaker?

    a. Evaluate the pacemaker in terms of efficiency and proper function.
    b. Attempt to repair or adjust the device.
    c. This patient must not receive any treatment.
    d. This patient must be treated just as if he or she didn't have a pacemaker.

35. Proper emergency care rendered to a COPD patient should include:

    a. assisting the patient to take his nitroglycerin.
    b. having the patient breathe into a paper bag.
    c. administering oxygen using a 24 percent venturi mask.
    d. administering oxygen using a non-rebreathing face mask at a flow rate of 10 LPM.

36. When transporting an unconscious CVA patient:

    a. transport in a semireclining position.
    b. place the patient on his or her back with the legs flexed at the knees.
    c. transport in a lateral recumbent position with the affected limbs underneath the patient.
    d. apply a cervical collar and secure the patient to a long spine board.

37. In cases of apparent child poisoning, with symptoms of nausea, the EMT should suspect:

    a. poison sumac.
    b. poison oak.
    c. apple blossoms.
    d. rhododendron.

38. To treat the victim of an injected poison, the EMT should:

    a. pull out stingers and venom sacs.
    b. scrape away stingers and venom sacs.
    c. apply a mud pack to remove the stinger and venom sac.
    d. leave the stinger and venom sac in place for the emergency department to deal with.

39. The proper dosage of syrup of ipecac to be given to a child under the age of 10 is:

    a. 1 teaspoon.
    b. 1 tablespoon.
    c. 2 teaspoons.
    d. 2 tablespoons.

40. Ingestion of which poisonous substance can result in burning of the mouth, throat, and stomach, "garlic breath," and vomiting?

    a. iodine.
    b. lye.
    c. chloroform.
    d. arsenic.

41. When treating a snake bite victim, the EMT should immediately:

    a. apply a constricting band above and below the fang marks.
    b. place an ice pack on the bite.
    c. cut into the bite and attempt to squeeze or suction the venom.
    d. apply a constricting band on either side of a joint.

42. The personnel at poison control centers:

    a. provide information only for cases of ingested poison.
    b. are usually available to give directions during the hours of 9 AM to 5 PM.
    c. provide information for all types of poisoning.
    d. publish guides and charts for poison control care that are distributed to EMS personnel to assist them in cases of emergency poisoning.

43. Proper emergency care for conscious victims of ingested poisoning includes:

    a. diluting and calling poison control.
    b. diluting and inducing vomiting.
    c. calling poison control and following their directions.
    d. inducing vomiting, then calling poison control.

44. The initial dose of ipecac and water may be repeated if the patient has not vomited in:

    a. 15 to 20 minutes.
    b. 30 minutes.
    c. 10 minutes.
    d. the EMT may not administer additional doses.

45. If the victim of ingested poisoning has been convulsing and is not fully conscious, the EMT should:

    a. dilute, then call poison control.
    b. induce vomiting, then call poison control.
    c. transport as soon as possible and call poison control en route.
    d. administer activated charcoal.

46. If you suspect your patient has inhaled a poisonous industrial compound, before you transport you should first:

    a. use protective clothing and breathing apparatus.
    b. provide care for the patient, even though the atmosphere is poisonous since the patient may die without your immediate aid.
    c. contact the hospital requesting assistance.
    d. call poison control before moving the patient.

47. Volatile chemicals that are sniffed or inhaled may act upon the central nervous system as:

    a. stimulants.
    b. depressants.
    c. hallucinogens.
    d. amphetamines.

48. The proper dosage of syrup of ipecac to induce vomiting in most cases of ingested poisoning for a conscious adult is:

    a. 4 tablespoons of ipecac mixed vigorously in 8 ounces of water.
    b. 2 tablespoons of ipecac followed by at least 8 ounces of water.
    c. 1 tablespoon of ipecac followed by 1 cup of water.
    d. 3 tablespoon of ipecac followed by several glasses of warm water.

49. As an EMT, your first step in the emergency care of a patient with a dry chemical acting as an absorbed poison will be to:

    a. remove all contaminated clothing.
    b. remove all jewelry and watches.
    c. brush the dry chemical away with something other than your hand.
    d. use water to flood all areas of the patient's body that have been exposed to the poison.

## SITUATIONS FOR FURTHER DISCUSSION

1. You have been called to treat a patient who appears slightly cyanotic, has a rapid pulse, rales, and swelling in the lower extremities.

    a. What do your primary and secondary surveys indicate the problem to be?
    b. What factors allow you to come to this conclusion?
    c. What factors caused you to rule out other conditions?
    d. What is the correct emergency treatment for this patient and in what order?
    e. In what position will you transport this patient?
    f. What continuing care will you provide for this patient en route to the hospital?
    g. What common allied problems might you expect to find or see develop with this patient's condition?
    h. What is the urgency of transportation to the hospital for this patient?

**86** MEDICAL EMERGENCIES SECTION ONE

    i. What would be your radio report to the hospital regarding the situation and present condition of the patient?

**2.** You respond to a call for a man not breathing. When you arrive, you find a pacemaker patient in cardiac arrest.

    a. What do your primary and secondary surveys indicate the problem to be?

    b. What factors allow you to come to this conclusion?

    c. What factors caused you to rule out other conditions?

    d. What is the correct emergency treatment for this patient and in what order?

    e. In what position will you transport this patient?

    f. What continuing care will you provide for this patient en route to the hospital?

    g. What common allied problems might you expect to find or see develop with this patient's condition?

    h. What is the urgency of transportation to the hospital for this patient?

    i. What would be your radio report to the hospital regarding the situation and present condition of the patient?

**3.** A 68-year-old man is found with a rapid, irregular pulse, normal blood pressure, and rapid breathing in puffs through pursed lips. There is also a wheezing sound when he breathes.

    a. What do your primary and secondary surveys indicate the problem to be?

    b. What factors allow you to come to this conclusion?

c. What factors caused you to rule out other conditions?

d. What is the correct emergency treatment for this patient and in what order?

e. In what position will you transport this patient?

f. What continuing care will you provide for this patient en route to the hospital?

g. What common allied problems might you expect to find or see develop with this patient's condition?

h. What is the urgency of transportation to the hospital for this patient?

i. What would be your radio report to the hospital regarding the situation and present condition of the patient?

4. A hysterical woman at a car accident appears uninjured, but she is breathing rapidly and complains of tingling in the upper extremities and cramping in the fingers of her left hand.

   a. What do your primary and secondary surveys indicate the problem to be?

   b. What factors allow you to come to this conclusion?

   c. What factors caused you to rule out other conditions?

   d. What is the correct emergency treatment for this patient and in what order?

   e. In what position will you transport this patient?

   f. What continuing care will you provide for this patient en route to the hospital?

## 88 MEDICAL EMERGENCIES SECTION ONE

g. What common allied problems might you expect to find or see develop with this patient's condition?

h. What is the urgency of transportation to the hospital for this patient?

i. What would be your radio report to the hospital regarding the situation and present condition of the patient?

5. You have been dispatched to a call involving a small child who was playing in a garage. The child is found semiconscious with a strange odor on his breath. Several open containers are nearby but most do not have labels.

   a. What do your primary and secondary surveys indicate the problem to be?

   b. What factors allow you to come to this conclusion?

   c. What factors caused you to rule out other conditions?

d. What is the correct emergency treatment for this patient and in what order?

e. In what position will you transport this patient?

f. What continuing care will you provide for this patient en route to the hospital?

g. What common allied problems might you expect to find or see develop with this patient's condition?

h. What is the urgency of transportation to the hospital for this patient?

i. What would be your radio report to the hospital regarding the situation and present condition of the patient?

## MEDICAL EMERGENCIES SECTION ONE 89

6. A woman who was working in the garden was stung by several bees. By the time you arrive, her face appears swollen and she feels a tightness across her chest. Several stingers are still stuck into her skin on her left arm.

   a. What do your primary and secondary surveys indicate the problem to be?

   b. What factors allow you to come to this conclusion?

   c. What factors caused you to rule out other conditions?

   d. What is the correct emergency treatment for this patient and in what order?

   e. In what position will you transport this patient?

   f. What continuing care will you provide for this patient en route to the hospital?

   g. What common allied problems might you expect to find or see develop with this patient's condition?

   h. What is the urgency of transportation to the hospital for this patient?

   i. What would be your radio report to the hospital regarding the situation and present condition of the patient?

7. A policeman suddenly feels dizzy while directing traffic around a chemical tanker truck accident site.

   a. What do your primary and secondary surveys indicate the problem to be?

   b. What factors allow you to come to this conclusion?

   c. What factors caused you to rule out other conditions?

## 90 MEDICAL EMERGENCIES SECTION ONE

d. What is the correct emergency treatment for this patient and in what order?

e. In what position will you transport this patient?

f. What continuing care will you will provide for this patient en route to the hospital?

g. What common allied problems might you expect to find or see develop with this patient's condition?

h. What is the urgency of transportation to the hospital for this patient?

i. What would be your radio report to the hospital regarding the situation and present condition of the patient?

# 14

# Medical Emergencies

## SECTION TWO: MEDICAL EMERGENCIES

- *Diabetes Mellitus*
- *Epilepsy and Other Convulsive Disorders*
- *Acute Abdominal Distress*
- *Communicable Diseases*
- *Alcohol and Substance Abuse*

---

1. When a diabetic takes too much insulin, has reduced his sugar intake by not eating, or has overexercised or exerted himself, the result is usually:

    a. diabetic shock.
    b. insulin shock.
    c. diabetic coma.
    d. insulin coma.

2. When not enough insulin is produced by the body, or the individual is not taking effective doses of insulin, this eventually will lead to:

    a. diabetic shock.
    b. insulin shock.
    c. diabetic coma.
    d. insulin coma.

3. Insulin shock occurs:

    a. when there is a decreased insulin supply.
    b. when there is a decreased oxygen supply.
    c. when there is too much insulin in the blood.
    d. as an allergic reaction.

4. The general signs and symptoms of an acute abdomen can include:

    a. pain, constipation, elevated blood pressure, distention of the abdomen, rigid abdomen.
    b. nausea, vomiting; slow pulse; rapid, shallow breathing; tenderness; abdominal wall spasms.
    c. diarrhea, high blood pressure, fever, soft abdomen, obvious protrusions, slow pulse.
    d. nausea, deep respirations, rapid pulse, rigid abdomen.

5. Whenever the EMT is in doubt as to whether a conscious patient is suffering from a decreased insulin supply or from an overabundance of insulin, the EMT should:

    a. transport immediately.
    b. have the patient breathe into a paper bag.
    c. administer sugar.
    d. administer insulin.

6. The noticeable distention of the abdomen caused by the accumulation of excess fluids is known as:

    a. acute abdomen.
    b. ascites.
    c. periosteum.
    d. peritonitis.

7. In order for glucose to pass from the bloodstream to the body cells:

   a. adduction must take place.
   b. insulin must be present.
   c. ketoacidosis must be adequate.
   d. insulin must not be present.

8. Diabetic coma results from:

   a. too much insulin in the blood.
   b. a decreased insulin supply.
   c. allergic reactions.
   d. lack of oxygen.

9. Emergency care for convulsive disorders includes:

   a. protecting the patient from injury.
   b. trying to hold the patient still.
   c. placing a bite stick in the patient's mouth to prevent the patient from biting his or her tongue.
   d. restraining the patient to prevent injury and inserting a bite stick.

10. The alcoholic patient may experience hallucinations and delerium tremens caused by:

    a. withdrawal.
    b. overdose.
    c. COPD.
    d. mixing alcohol and drugs.

11. Which of the following causes nervous system stimulation?

    a. Barbiturates
    b. Amphetamines
    c. Codeine
    d. LSD

12. A commonly abused narcotic resulting in reduced pulse, lowered skin temperature, and constricted pupils is:

    a. cocaine.
    b. methaqualone.
    c. mescaline.
    d. heroin.

13. The chemical PCP is a:

    a. depressant.
    b. mind-affecting drug.
    c. volatile chemical.
    d. barbiturate.

14. When providing emergency care for drug abuse patients:

    a. it is not necessary to perform a secondary survey.
    b. do not talk to the patient, since your questions may annoy the patient.
    c. transport the patient as soon as possible, and monitor vitals while remaining alert for convulsions and vomiting.
    d. restrain the patient and transport even if he or she refuses treatment.

## SITUATIONS FOR FURTHER DISCUSSION

1. You find an unconscious male wearing medic-alert identification indicating a diabetic problem. The pulse appears rapid, blood pressure is normal. The skin appears cool and clammy. There are no signs of injury.

   a. What do your primary and secondary surveys indicate the problem to be?

   b. What factors allow you to come to this conclusion?

   c. What factors caused you to rule out other conditions?

   d. What is the correct emergency treatment for this patient and in what order?

MEDICAL EMERGENCIES SECTION TWO   93

e. In what position will you transport this patient?

f. What continuing care will you provide for this patient en route to the hospital?

g. What common allied problems might you expect to find or see develop with this patient's condition?

h. What is the urgency of transportation to the hospital for this patient?

i. What would be your radio report to the hospital regarding the situation and present condition of the patient?

2. You respond to a seizure call and find family members holding down a writhing patient while trying to force a spoon into the patient's mouth.

   a. What do your primary and secondary surveys indicate the problem to be?

b. What factors allow you to come to this conclusion?

c. What factors caused you to rule out other conditions?

d. What is the correct emergency treatment for this patient and in what order?

e. In what position will you transport this patient?

f. What continuing care will you provide for this patient en route to the hospital?

g. What common allied problems might you expect to find or see develop with this patient's condition?

h. What is the urgency of transportation to the hospital for this patient?

# 94 MEDICAL EMERGENCIES SECTION TWO

    i. What would be your radio report to the hospital regarding the situation and present condition of the patient?

3. While questioning a suspected drug abuse patient who is drifting in and out of consciousness about what was taken, the patient is reluctant to tell you anything because the police are present.

    a. What do your primary and secondary surveys indicate the problem to be?

    b. What factors allow you to come to this conclusion?

    c. What factors caused you to rule out other conditions?

    d. What is the correct emergency treatment for this patient and in what order?

    e. In what position will you transport this patient?

    f. What continuing care will you provide for this patient en route to the hospital?

    g. What common allied problems might you expect to find or see develop with this patient's condition?

    h. What is the urgency of transportation to the hospital for this patient?

    i. What would be your radio report to the hospital regarding the situation and present condition of the patient?

# 15

# Pediatric Emergencies

• *Infants and Children—Special Patients*

---

1. When providing emergency care for a child:

   a. do not allow the child to bring along a toy, which may be contaminated.
   b. conduct the patient survey and interview at a rapid pace, in order to get it over with as quickly as possible.
   c. always assure the child that everything is fine; let him or her deal with the truth later.
   d. always tell the child what you are going to do as you take vital signs and perform a physical examination.

2. The normal pulse rate of an infant who is 6 months old is:

   a. 140 to 150 beats per minute.
   b. 120 beats per minute.
   c. 110 beats per minute.
   d. 100 beats per minute.

3. When performing CPR on an infant, the proper depth of compression is:

   a. ½ to ¾ inch.
   b. ½ to 1 inch.
   c. 1 to 1½ inches.
   d. 1½ to 2 inches.

4. The EMT should care for children who are poisoning victims by following the advice of:

   a. instructions and antidotes on the container.
   b. advice from the parents.
   c. the local poison control center.
   d. your own classroom experience of poisonings and antidotes.

5. A person is considered to be a child between the ages of:

   a. 1 year to 8 years.
   b. 15 months to 10 years.
   c. 18 months to 12 years.
   d. 2 years to 8 years.

6. The EMT should consider an infant to be in shock if blood loss is:

   a. 100 ml or more.
   b. 25 ml or more.
   c. 50 ml or more.
   d. 80 ml or more.

7. To determine whether or not a two-year-old child has a pulse, the EMT should palpate for the:

   a. apical pulse.
   b. brachial pulse.
   c. carotid pulse.
   d. radial pulse.

8. The EMT should treat a child with an impaled fishhook by:

   a. pulling free the fishhook.
   b. pushing the point through the skin and cutting off the barb.
   c. following the curve of the hook and pulling it through.
   d. transporting the child to a medical facility without removing the fishhook.

## 96 PEDIATRIC EMERGENCIES

9. The EMT must transport a child between the ages of 1 and 5 years of age if the child has an oral temperature above:

   a. 100 degrees.
   b. 103 degrees.
   c. 101 degrees.
   d. 98.6 degrees.

10. What is the normal breathing rate for a child between the ages of 2 and 4 years?

    a. 46
    b. 25
    c. 20
    d. 12

11. CPR compressions on an 8-year-old child are applied using:

    a. the tips of 2 or 3 fingers.
    b. the heels of both hands.
    c. the tips of 4 fingers.
    d. the heel of one hand.

12. As a result of a "bike fork compression" injury, the body part that is usually injured is the:

    a. elbow.
    b. shoulder.
    c. ankle.
    d. chest.

13. Appropriate actions by an EMT caring for a baby who has suffered Sudden Infant Death Syndrome include:

    a. questioning the parents to be sure they did not contribute to the death.
    b. providing basic life support measures.
    c. not transporting the possible SIDS victim until the police have completed their investigation.
    d. informing the parents, as gently as possible, of the infant's death.

14. The EMT must consider an 8-year-old child to be in shock if blood loss is greater than:

    a. 200 ml.
    b. 500 ml.
    c. 1000 ml.
    d. 1500 ml.

15. When attempting to remove a ring from a child's swollen finger, the EMT may try to slide the ring off after lubricating the finger with:

    a. water.
    b. heating oil.
    c. motor oil.
    d. petroleum lubricating oil.

16. If you suspect an injured child to be the victim of child abuse, as an EMT you should:

    a. ask the child if he or she has been abused.
    b. let the parents know that you are suspicious.
    c. mind your own business.
    d. report your suspicions to the emergency department staff.

17. Infants are considered to be between the ages of birth and:

    a. 1 year.
    b. 15 months.
    c. 18 months.
    d. 2 years.

18. The normal systolic blood pressure of a 6-month-old infant should be:

    a. 30 mmHg.
    b. 50 mmHg.
    c. 70 mmHg.
    d. 90 mmHg.

19. When attempting to clear the airway of a conscious 4-year-old child suffering an airway obstruction, the EMT should:

    a. administer 6 abdominal thrusts.
    b. administer 4 chest thrusts.
    c. perform finger sweeps.
    d. attempt to ventilate.

20. In an effort to cool a child with a high fever, the EMT may:

    a. sponge the child with alcohol.
    b. cover the child with a towel that has been saturated with tepid water.
    c. submerge the child in a tub of ice water.
    d. cover the child with a towel that has been saturated with ice water.

## SITUATIONS FOR FURTHER DISCUSSION

1. You are called by a distraught parent whose child has a small ring stuck on her finger. The finger is swollen and tender. Vital signs appear normal and no other injuries are evident.

   a. What do your primary and secondary surveys indicate the problem to be?

   b. What factors allow you to come to this conclusion?

   c. What factors caused you to rule out other conditions?

   d. What is the correct emergency treatment for this patient and in what order?

   e. In what position will you transport this patient?

   f. What continuing care will you provide for this patient en route to the hospital?

   g. What common allied problems might you expect to find or see develop with this patient's condition?

   h. What is the urgency of transportation to the hospital for this patient?

   i. What would be your radio report to the hospital regarding the situation and present condition of the patient?

2. A three-year-old child is found to have a rectal temperature of 103 degrees. The parents have been sponging the child with an alcohol/water solution for the past hour. The child appears to be shivering despite her high body temperature.

   a. What do your primary and secondary surveys indicate the problem to be?

   b. What factors allow you to come to this conclusion?

   c. What factors caused you to rule out other conditions?

## 98  PEDIATRIC EMERGENCIES

d. What is the correct emergency treatment for this patient and in what order?

e. In what position will you transport this patient?

f. What continuing care will you provide for this patient en route to the hospital?

g. What common allied problems might you expect to find or see develop with this patient's condition?

h. What is the urgency of transportation to the hospital for this patient?

i. What would be your radio report to the hospital regarding the situation and present condition of the patient?

3. You are called to treat a 4-year-old child who is suspected of having ingested some of his mother's pills. The parent isn't sure what or how much may have been taken. The child appears to drift in and out of consciousness and the eyes appear to roll back.

a. What do your primary and secondary surveys indicate the problem to be?

b. What factors allow you to come to this conclusion?

c. What factors caused you to rule out other conditions?

d. What is the correct emergency treatment for this patient and in what order?

e. In what position will you transport this patient?

PEDIATRIC EMERGENCIES   99

f. What continuing care will you provide for this patient en route to the hospital?

g. What common allied problems might you expect to find or see develop with this patient's condition?

h. What is the urgency of transportation to the hospital for this patient?

i. What would be your radio report to the hospital regarding the situation and present condition of the patient?

# 16

# Childbirth

- *Childbirth*
- *Normal Delivery*
- *Complications*
- *Predelivery Emergencies*
- *Abnormal Deliveries*

---

1. The unborn, developing human organism is called:
   a. an infant.
   b. a fetus.
   c. a baby.
   d. premature.

2. The first stage of labor starts with contractions and ends when the:
   a. fetus enters the birth canal.
   b. cervix is fully dilated.
   c. baby is born.
   d. afterbirth is born.

3. If the head of the baby is still enclosed in the amniotic sac, the EMT should:
   a. allow the delivery to continue.
   b. suction the amniotic sac.
   c. transport immediately to the hospital.
   d. use your finger to puncture the membrane and remove it from the area of the baby's mouth and nose.

4. Contractions every 2 or 3 minutes are a usual sign that birth is imminent. However, a prolonged delivery is indicated and the mother must be transported without delay if the body is not delivered within:
   a. 10 minutes.
   b. 20 minutes.
   c. 30 minutes.
   d. 45 minutes.

5. The developing fetus grows in the mother's:
   a. uterus.
   b. cervix.
   c. vulva.
   d. vagina.

6. Your patient is a young woman about to have her third child. Her contractions are 2 minutes apart, and she is crowning. You should:
   a. prepare for immediate transport.
   b. prepare for an imminent birth.
   c. allow the mother to go to the bathroom to move her bowels.
   d. hold the mother's legs together.

7. If bleeding continues from the umbilical cord after cutting, the EMT should:
   a. untie or unclamp the cord and replace the tie or clamp.
   b. attempt to adjust the clamp or retie the knot.
   c. transport immediately.
   d. apply another tie or clamp as close to the original one as possible.

8. If a woman in labor begins to bleed excessively from the vagina, you should:
   a. place the patient in a lateral recumbent position and treat for shock.
   b. hold the patient's legs together.
   c. place a sterile dressing in the vagina.
   d. apply direct pressure to the abdomen.

9. The neck of the uterus is called the:
   a. crown.
   b. vagina.
   c. cervix.
   d. womb.

10. To assist in delivering the baby's upper shoulder, gently:
    a. guide the baby's head upward.
    b. support the baby's head.
    c. guide the baby's head downward.
    d. pull on the baby's head.

11. Mother and newborn are doing well and there are no respiratory problems or uncontrolled bleeding. While awaiting delivery of the placenta, you may delay transportation to the hospital for up to:
    a. 20 minutes.
    b. 30 minutes.
    c. 40 minutes.
    d. Do not delay, transport immediately.

12. When providing oxygen to the newborn, the EMT should:
    a. blow the stream of oxygen directly into the baby's face.
    b. deliver the oxygen into the top of an aluminum foil tent placed over the baby's head.
    c. use a pressure-cycled resuscitator.
    d. never administer oxygen to a newborn infant since this could cause blindness.

13. The birth canal is called the:
    a. cervix.
    b. umbilicus.
    c. vulva.
    d. vagina.

14. When your evaluation leads you to believe that birth is imminent, you should prepare by placing the mother:
    a. at the edge of the bed with her legs dangling over the side.
    b. on a blanket on the floor.
    c. in a large, comfortable chair.
    d. in the center of the bed, leaving yourself 2 feet below her legs.

15. The advanced stage of toxemia of pregnancy, which can lead to convulsions and coma, is called:
    a. placenta previa.
    b. abrupt placenta.
    c. eclampsia.
    d. ectopic pregnancy.

16. The exchange of oxygen and wastes occurs between the mother and the developing fetus in the:
    a. placenta.
    b. uterus.
    c. cervix.
    d. amniotic sac.

17. To care for a newborn who is still attached to the placenta, the EMT should first:
    a. place the baby on the mother's abdomen.
    b. place the baby on the bed.
    c. lift the baby by its feet and slap its bottom.
    d. place the baby below the level of the mother's vagina.

18. As you prepare to cut the umbilical cord, apply the first clamp or tie to the cord approximately:
    a. 6 inches from the baby.
    b. 10 inches from the baby.
    c. 6 inches from the mother.
    d. 10 inches from the mother.

19. Which type of pregnancy may cause women to have acute abdominal pain; rapid, weak pulse; slight vaginal bleeding; and go into shock?
    a. Eclampsic
    b. Toxemic
    c. Ectopic
    d. Extruded

20. During normal childbirth, the placenta is expelled:
    a. before the baby is born.
    b. after the baby is born.
    c. with the baby as it is born.
    d. at no specified time.

21. A newborn infant should begin breathing within:
    a. 10 seconds.
    b. 20 seconds.

c. 30 seconds.
d. 45 seconds.

22. A spontaneous abortion is the term given to describe a miscarriage that occurs before the:

    a. 12th week of pregnancy.
    b. 16th week of pregnancy.
    c. 24th week of pregnancy.
    d. 28th week of pregnancy.

23. The developing fetus is enclosed in a thin, membraneous tissue known as the:

    a. umbilicus.
    b. placenta.
    c. amniotic sac.
    d. uterus.

24. To encourage a newborn infant to breathe, the EMT should:

    a. deliver several chest compressions.
    b. snap your index finger against the soles of the baby's feet.
    c. administer oxygen.
    d. lift the baby by its feet and slap its bottom.

25. The skin between the vulva and anus is known as the:

    a. peritoneum.
    b. perineum.
    c. sacrum.
    d. vagina.

26. During a breech delivery, it may be necessary to place your gloved hand carefully into the vagina to assure an open airway if the head does not deliver within:

    a. 4 minutes.
    b. 3 minutes.
    c. 10 minutes.
    d. 20 minutes.

27. A prolapsed umbilical cord means that the cord:

    a. is wrapped around the baby's neck.
    b. the cord does not have a pulse.
    c. the cord presents first.
    d. is no longer attached to the baby.

28. Crowning occurs when the:

    a. baby's head has been delivered.
    b. cervix is dilated 10 centimeters.
    c. bag of waters breaks.
    d. presenting part of the baby first bulges from the vaginal opening.

29. The newborn should be positioned on its:

    a. side with the head positioned slightly lower than its body.
    b. back with the head in the upright position.
    c. side with the head positioned slightly higher than its body.
    d. back with the head turned to the side.

30. The EMT may control vaginal bleeding after delivery by:

    a. carefully placing sterile dressings inside the vagina.
    b. applying direct pressure firmly on the abdomen for 10 to 30 minutes.
    c. massage the mother's lower abdomen with a slight circular motion.
    d. using the femoral artery pressure point.

31. If you find an upper or lower limb presenting during evaluation of the mother you should:

    a. pull gently but firmly on the limb.
    b. replace the limb in the vagina.
    c. place your hand in the vagina.
    d. transport immediately to the hospital.

32. Normal headfirst birth is called a:

    a. cephalic delivery.
    b. breech delivery.
    c. ectopic delivery.
    d. prolapsed delivery.

33. An infant's skull contains fontanelles, which are:

    a. blood vessels.
    b. bones.
    c. soft spots.
    d. rigid membranes.

34. If the EMT cannot detect a brachial pulse in a non-breathing newborn, the EMT should:

    a. begin CPR.
    b. cut the cord, then begin CPR.
    c. clamp the cord, then begin CPR.
    d. clamp and cut the cord, then begin CPR.

35. A newborn is considered to be premature if it is born before the:

    a. 9th month of pregnancy.
    b. expected due date.
    c. 5th month of pregnancy.
    d. 7th month of pregnancy.

**36.** If the buttocks or both feet of the baby deliver first, the birth is called a:

a. cephalic delivery.
b. posterior delivery.
c. breech birth.
d. limb presentation.

**37.** Suctioning the mouth and nose of the newborn is accomplished by using:

a. finger sweeps.
b. a rubber bulb syringe.
c. a portable suction unit.
d. an oropharyngeal airway.

**38.** The rate for pulmonary resuscitation of the newborn is:

a. one breath every 3 seconds.
b. one breath every 5 seconds.
c. two breaths every 5 seconds.
d. two breaths every 10 seconds.

**39.** Special care in the treatment of a premature infant includes:

a. holding the baby up by the feet and slapping its bottom.
b. blowing a stream of oxygen directly on the baby's face.
c. transporting in a warm ambulance.
d. removing all umbilical clamps if bleeding is evident.

**40.** The third stage of labor begins when:

a. the fetus enters the birth canal.
b. crowning occurs.
c. the baby is born.
d. the placenta is delivered.

**41.** If you cannot loosen and reposition an umbilical cord that is wrapped around the baby's neck, you should:

a. delay delivery and transport to the hospital.
b. allow the delivery to continue.
c. pull firmly on the cord until you are able to loosen and reposition it.
d. clamp the cord in 2 places and cut it between the two clamps.

**42.** The average time in labor for a woman having her first baby is usually:

a. 16 to 17 hours.
b. 11 to 12 hours.
c. 5 to 6 hours.
d. 22 to 24 hours.

**43.** After the placenta is delivered, the EMT should:

a. dispose of it at the scene.
b. examine the placenta and other tissues for completeness before disposing of them.
c. save the placental tissues in newspaper to be disposed of at the hospital.
d. save all placental tissues in a plastic bag and transport with the mother to the hospital.

**44.** The proper ratio of compressions to breaths during newborn CPR is:

a. 15 to 2.
b. 3 to 1.
c. 5 to 2.
d. 5 to 1.

## SITUATIONS FOR FURTHER DISCUSSION

**1.** You are called to assist with a delivery and find a 30-year-old woman who is full term and experiencing contractions that are 5 minutes apart. Her husband tells you that this will be their third child. The woman feels a need to move her bowels and asks you to help her get to the bathroom.

a. What do your primary and secondary surveys indicate the problem to be?

b. What factors allow you to come to this conclusion?

c. What factors caused you to rule out other conditions?

**104  CHILDBIRTH**

d. What is the correct emergency treatment for this patient and in what order?

e. In what position will you transport this patient?

f. What continuing care will you provide for this patient en route to the hospital?

g. What common allied problems might you expect to find or see develop with this patient's condition?

h. What is the urgency of transportation to the hospital for this patient?

i. What would be your radio report to the hospital regarding the situation and present condition of the patient?

2. A 27-year-old woman in her seventh month of pregnancy calls you because she is experiencing contractions and has a bloody show. The contractions are 5 minutes apart.

a. What do your primary and secondary surveys indicate the problem to be?

b. What factors allow you to come to this conclusion?

c. What factors caused you to rule out other conditions?

d. What is the correct emergency treatment for this patient and in what order?

e. In what position will you transport this patient?

f. What continuing care will you provide for this patient en route to the hospital?

g. What common allied problems might you expect to find or see develop with this patient's condition?

h. What is the urgency of transportation to the hospital for this patient?

i. What would be your radio report to the hospital regarding the situation and present condition of the patient?

3. Visual inspection of a woman who is full term indicates the umbilical cord protruding from the vagina. The woman is experiencing contractions every 3 minutes.

   a. What do your primary and secondary surveys indicate the problem to be?

   b. What factors allow you to come to this conclusion?

   c. What factors caused you to rule out other conditions?

   d. What is the correct emergency treatment for this patient and in what order?

e. In what position will you transport this patient?

f. What continuing care will you provide for this patient en route to the hospital?

g. What common allied problems might you expect to find or see develop with this patient's condition?

h. What is the urgency of transportation to the hospital for this patient?

i. What would be your radio report to the hospital regarding the situation and present condition of the patient?

4. After delivery of a healthy baby, the placenta has not delivered within 20 minutes.

   a. What do your primary and secondary surveys indicate the problem to be?

## 106 CHILDBIRTH

b. What factors allow you to come to this conclusion?

c. What factors caused you to rule out other conditions?

d. What is the correct emergency treatment for this patient and in what order?

e. In what position will you transport this patient?

f. What continuing care will you provide for this patient en route to the hospital?

g. What common allied problems might you expect to find or see develop with this patient's condition?

h. What is the urgency of transportation to the hospital for this patient?

i. What would be your radio report to the hospital regarding the situation and present condition of the patient?

5. A woman has just delivered a healthy baby, but she still is experiencing contractions.

   a. What do your primary and secondary surveys indicate the problem to be?

   b. What factors allow you to come to this conclusion?

   c. What factors caused you to rule out other conditions?

   d. What is the correct emergency treatment for this patient and in what order?

   e. In what position will you transport this patient?

f. What continuing care will you provide for this patient en route to the hospital?

g. What common allied problems might you expect to find or see develop with this patient's condition?

h. What is the urgency of transportation to the hospital for this patient?

i. What would be your radio report to the hospital regarding the situation and present condition of the patient?

6. When you inspect a pregnant woman for signs of crowning, you find the presenting part to be the buttocks. The contractions are 2 minutes apart and the bag of waters has broken.

   a. What do your primary and secondary surveys indicate the problem to be?

   b. What factors allow you to come to this conclusion?

   c. What factors caused you to rule out other conditions?

   d. What is the correct emergency treatment for this patient and in what order?

   e. In what position will you transport this patient?

   f. What continuing care will you provide for this patient en route to the hospital?

   g. What common allied problems might you expect to find or see develop with this patient's condition?

   h. What is the urgency of transportation to the hospital for this patient?

   i. What would be your radio report to the hospital regarding the situation and present condition of the patient?

# 17

# Burns and Hazardous Materials

- *Environmental Factors*
- *Burns*
- *Injuries Due to Electricity*
- *Hazardous Materials*
- *Radiation Accidents*
- *Explosions*

---

1. The source of a thermal burn can be:

    a. flame.
    b. acids.
    c. AC current.
    d. ultraviolet rays.

2. Critical burns are:

    a. second-degree burns covering 12 percent of the body surface.
    b. all burns complicated by injuries of the respiratory tract, soft tissues, and bones.
    c. second-degree burns involving 25 percent of the body surface.
    d. third-degree burns involving 9 percent of the body surface.

3. The type of burn characterized by deep, intense pain, reddening, blisters, and a mottled appearance to the skin is called a:

    a. first-degree burn.
    b. second-degree burn.
    c. third-degree burn.
    d. fourth-degree burn.

4. Electrical burns can be caused by:

    a. various caustic chemicals.
    b. ultraviolet light.
    c. lightning.
    d. radioactive sources.

5. The most serious effect of electric shock usually is:

    a. the burn.
    b. convulsions.
    c. disrupted nerve pathways.
    d. respiratory and/or cardiac arrest.

6. To establish a safe zone at the scene of a hazardous materials accident, the EMT should:

    a. stay downwind from the site of the accident.
    b. stay downhill from the accident site.
    c. set up position in a low-lying area.
    d. avoid placing him- or herself higher than the accident scene.

7. A burn involving only the outermost layer of the epidermis is classified as:

    a. first-degree.
    b. second-degree.
    c. third-degree.
    d. fourth-degree.

BURNS AND HAZARDOUS MATERIALS   109

8. With which type of burn does the patient rarely feel pain and is the burn usually charred black or with areas that are dry and white?

   a. Mild partial thickness burn
   b. First-degree
   c. Second-degree
   d. Third-degree

9. Using the "Rule of Nines," what percentage of an infant's body is involved if the head, neck, chest, and abdomen are burned?

   a. 9 percent
   b. 18 percent
   c. 27 percent
   d. 36 percent

10. Which radiation particles are high in energy level and cannot be stopped by heavy clothing?

    a. Alpha
    b. Beta
    c. Gamma
    d. X-ray

11. To care for extensive first-, second-, and third-degree burns, the EMT should:

    a. apply burn ointment liberally.
    b. flood the affected area with a copious flow of water.
    c. wrap the patient in a clean, dry sheet.
    d. apply soap and water to clean the area of the burn.

12. When treating a victim of smoke inhalation, the EMT's priority is:

    a. airway patency.
    b. treatment for shock.
    c. transportation.
    d. care for eye irritations.

13. Using the "Rule of Nines," what percentage of an adult's body is involved if the head, neck, one entire arm, and front of one leg are burned?

    a. 9 percent
    b. 18 percent
    c. 27 percent
    d. 36 percent

14. The first priority of care at the scene of an explosion is:

    a. basic life support.
    b. a complete patient assessment.
    c. internal bleeding.
    d. contusions to the lungs.

15. Proper care for chemical burns to the eye includes:

    a. use of a neutralizing chemical.
    b. not forcing the patient's eyes open.
    c. washing the eye with a flow of water.
    d. not covering the eye after washing.

16. The EMT's initial care in treating a patient with a chemical burn caused by dry lime is to:

    a. wash the chemical from the burn site using water.
    b. brush the dry lime from the patient's skin, hair, and clothing.
    c. flood the burn site with sterile saline solution.
    d. apply moist sterile dressings.

17. Second-degree burns involving 15 to 30 percent of the body surface are considered:

    a. critical.
    b. moderate.
    c. minor.
    d. life-threatening.

18. The EMT should cover electrical burns with:

    a. moist sterile dressings.
    b. dry sterile dressings.
    c. tin foil.
    d. plastic wrap.

## SITUATIONS FOR FURTHER DISCUSSION

1. While on standby at a major structure fire, a burn victim is brought to you by firefighters. The victim is a 40-year-old male who fell asleep while smoking. He appears to have suffered second- and third-degree burns over his torso (front and back), upper extremities, and head. The man also is in acute respiratory distress and has a rapid and weak pulse. A blood pressure cannot be taken due to extensive burns to his arms.

   a. What do your primary and secondary surveys indicate the problem to be?

   b. What factors allow you to come to this conclusion?

### 110  BURNS AND HAZARDOUS MATERIALS

   c. What factors caused you to rule out other conditions?

   d. What is the correct emergency treatment for this patient and in what order?

   e. In what position will you transport this patient?

   f. What continuing care will you provide for this patient en route to the hospital?

   g. What common allied problems might you expect to find or see develop with this patient's condition?

   h. What is the urgency of transportation to the hospital for this patient?

   i. What would be your radio report to the hospital regarding the situation and present condition of the patient?

2. A student in a chemistry lab explosion has had some unknown substance sprayed into his face, which is stinging his eyes.

   a. What do your primary and secondary surveys indicate the problem to be?

   b. What factors allow you to come to this conclusion?

   c. What factors caused you to rule out other conditions?

   d. What is the correct emergency treatment for this patient and in what order?

   e. In what position will you transport this patient?

   f. What continuing care will you provide for this patient en route to the hospital?

g. What common allied problems might you expect to find or see develop with this patient's condition?

h. What is the urgency of transportation to the hospital for this patient?

i. What would be your radio report to the hospital regarding the situation and present condition of the patient?

3. A telephone company worker is found lying motionless at the bottom of a ladder that is touching electrical wires overhead. His arm is still touching the ladder. A police officer at the scene has requested that the utility company turn off the power to that section of town. He now receives word that power has been turned off and tells you it is safe to move the patient.

   a. What do your primary and secondary surveys indicate the problem to be?

   b. What factors allow you to come to this conclusion?

   c. What factors caused you to rule out other conditions?

d. What is the correct emergency treatment for this patient and in what order?

e. In what position will you transport this patient?

f. What continuing care will you provide for this patient en route to the hospital?

g. What common allied problems might you expect to find or see develop with this patient's condition?

h. What is the urgency of transportation to the hospital for this patient?

i. What would be your radio report to the hospital regarding the situation and present condition of the patient?

## 112 BURNS AND HAZARDOUS MATERIALS

4. A tractor trailer truck carrying nuclear fuel for a local power plant is involved in an accident and the driver is trapped inside the tractor requiring extrication. No federal agencies are yet on the scene to confirm or manage any possible leak of radioactive material.

   a. What do your primary and secondary surveys indicate the problem to be?

   b. What factors allow you to come to this conclusion?

   c. What factors caused you to rule out other conditions?

   d. What is the correct emergency treatment for this patient and in what order?

   e. In what position will you transport this patient?

   f. What continuing care will you provide for this patient en route to the hospital?

   g. What common allied problems might you expect to find or see develop with this patient's condition?

   h. What is the urgency of transportation to the hospital for this patient?

   i. What would be your radio report to the hospital regarding the situation and present condition of the patient?

# 18

# Environmental Emergencies

## SECTION ONE: HEAT- AND COLD-RELATED EMERGENCIES

- *Emergencies Due to Excessive Heat*
- *Emergencies Due to Excessive Cold*

---

1. Initially, the skin of a person suffering from frostnip will be:
   a. white.
   b. red.
   c. waxy.
   d. bluish-gray.

2. Proper emergency care for heat cramps includes:
   a. administering salted water or commercial electrolyte fluids by mouth.
   b. removing enough clothing to cool the patient without chilling.
   c. cooling the patient rapidly, in any manner.
   d. placing cold packs in each armpit.

3. A condition that develops after the lower extremities have remained in water that is just above freezing for a prolonged period is:
   a. chilblains.
   b. trenchfoot.
   c. hypothermia.
   d. gangrene.

4. Which emergency, brought about by excessive exposure to heat, is a mild form of shock caused by blood pooling in the skin as the body attempts to rid itself of excess heat?
   a. Heat stroke
   b. Heat exhaustion
   c. Hypothermia
   d. Heat cramps

5. When caring for a patient with mild to moderate hypothermia, which should the EMT attend to first?
   a. Wrap the patient in blankets.
   b. Apply heat to the patient's body.
   c. Remove wet clothing.
   d. Administer warm liquids.

6. The EMT should consider any case of hypothermia to be very serious if the patient has:
   a. a core temperature below 95 degrees.
   b. intense, uncontrolled shivering.
   c. become unconscious.
   d. difficulty breathing.

113

**114** ENVIRONMENTAL EMERGENCIES SECTION ONE

7. The true emergency caused by the body's failure to sweat in response to a prolonged exposure to high ambient temperature is called:

    a. heat cramps.
    b. heat stroke.
    c. heat exhaustion.
    d. hypothermia.

8. Emergency care for rewarming a frozen extremity is:

    a. rubbing the frostbitten or frozen area gently with your warm hands.
    b. rubbing snow on the frostbitten or frozen area.
    c. placing the frozen part in a water bath with a temperature of 100 to 105 degrees Fahrenheit.
    d. rewarming the frozen part in a water bath with a temperature of 107 to 115 degrees Fahrenheit.

## SITUATIONS FOR FURTHER DISCUSSION

1. A man has collapsed while playing tennis on a hot and humid day. When you arrive, he feels hot to your touch and his armpits feel dry. His pulse is rapid and full, and he drifts in and out of consciousness.

    a. What do your primary and secondary surveys indicate the problem to be?

    b. What factors allow you to come to this conclusion?

    c. What factors caused you to rule out other conditions?

    d. What is the correct emergency treatment for this patient and in what order?

    e. In what position will you transport this patient?

    f. What continuing care will you provide for this patient en route to the hospital?

    g. What common allied problems might you expect to find or see develop with this patient's condition?

    h. What is the urgency of transportation to the hospital for this patient?

    i. What would be your radio report to the hospital regarding the situation and present condition of the patient?

2. A hiker who has been lost for three days during a snowstorm is found complaining of loss of sensation in both his feet and fingers.

    a. What do your primary and secondary surveys indicate the problem to be?

b. What factors allow you to come to this conclusion?

c. What factors caused you to rule out other conditions?

d. What is the correct emergency treatment for this patient and in what order?

e. In what position will you transport this patient?

f. What continuing care will you provide for this patient en route to the hospital?

g. What common allied problems might you expect to find or see develop with this patient's condition?

h. What is the urgency of transportation to the hospital for this patient?

i. What would be your radio report to the hospital regarding the situation and present condition of the patient?

# 18

# Environmental Emergencies

## SECTION TWO: WATER- AND ICE-RELATED ACCIDENTS

- *Accidents Involving Water*
- *Diving Accidents*
- *Accidents Involving Ice*

---

1. In all cases of water-related accidents, the EMT should suspect that the unconscious patient has:

   a. an airway obstruction.
   b. severe brain damage after 10 minutes.
   c. neck and spinal injuries.
   d. suffered cardiac arrest.

2. The EMT should not attempt a water rescue:

   a. unless he or she is a good swimmer and trained in water rescue.
   b. if he or she is alone.
   c. if the patient is unresponsive.
   d. unless a boat is available.

3. The onset of decompression sickness for scuba divers is usually:

   a. immediate, occurring even before the diver surfaces.
   b. obvious as soon as the diver surfaces.
   c. slow, taking from 1 to 48 hours to appear.
   d. avoided if the diver flies within 12 hours of a dive.

4. Pulmonary resuscitation should be initiated on water rescue victims:

   a. as soon as the patient is on land.
   b. in the water.
   c. only if no more than 10 minutes have elapsed.
   d. only if there is no water in the lungs.

5. If the EMT must work alone in attempting an ice rescue, he or she should:

   a. walk only on stable ice.
   b. leave a signal if he or she must enter the water.
   c. wear a PFD when he or she goes onto ice that is rapidly breaking.
   d. throw a rope or push a ladder to the victim.

### SITUATIONS FOR FURTHER DISCUSSION

1. You respond to a swimming pool diving accident where the lifeguards suspect spinal injury. The guards and several bystanders are supporting the victim in shallow water and are providing mouth-to-mouth resuscitation. The first EMT to reach the victim detects that there is no carotid pulse.

   a. What do your primary and secondary surveys indicate the problem to be?

b. What factors allow you to come to this conclusion?

c. What factors caused you to rule out other conditions?

d. What is the correct emergency treatment for this patient and in what order?

e. In what position will you transport this patient?

f. What continuing care will you provide for this patient en route to the hospital?

g. What common allied problems might you expect to find or see develop with this patient's condition?

h. What is the urgency of transportation to the hospital for this patient?

i. What would be your radio report to the hospital regarding the situation and present condition of the patient?

2. You are first to arrive at the scene of an accident in which a child has fallen through the ice. The child is visible, holding onto the edge of the break some 50 yards offshore. No one else has arrived yet.

   a. What do your primary and secondary surveys indicate the problem to be?

   b. What factors allow you to come to this conclusion?

   c. What factors caused you to rule out other conditions?

   d. What is the correct emergency treatment for this patient and in what order?

   e. In what position will you transport this patient?

**118** ENVIRONMENTAL EMERGENCIES SECTION TWO

    f. What continuing care will you provide for this patient en route to the hospital?

    g. What common allied problems might you expect to find or see develop with this patient's condition?

    h. What is the urgency of transportation to the hospital for this patient?

    i. What would be your radio report to the hospital regarding the situation and present condition of the patient?

**3.** A child has been pulled from the murky bottom of an abandoned swimming pool. The child is not breathing and has no pulse. Bystanders state that the child may have been under the water for at least 15 minutes. The water feels very cold to your touch.

    a. What do your primary and secondary surveys indicate the problem to be?

    b. What factors allow you to come to this conclusion?

    c. What factors caused you to rule out other conditions?

    d. What is the correct emergency treatment for this patient and in what order?

    e. In what position will you transport this patient?

    f. What continuing care will you provide for this patient en route to the hospital?

    g. What common allied problems might you expect to find or see develop with this patient's condition?

    h. What is the urgency of transportation to the hospital for this patient?

    i. What would be your radio report to the hospital regarding the situation and present condition of the patient?

# 19

# Special Patients and Behavioral Problems

- *The Management of Special Patients*
- *Behavioral Problems*
- *EMT Stress Syndrome*

---

1. When the EMT acts in a calm, professional manner while talking with and listening to a patient in order to provide emotional support, this is called:

   a. emotional emergency.
   b. personal interaction.
   c. interactive triage.
   d. patient concern.

2. When treating an elderly patient whose spouse or close friend is present, the EMT should:

   a. consider that the EMT has two patients.
   b. ask the spouse or close friend to wait in another room.
   c. not talk to or about the patient in front of the family.
   d. none of the above.

3. The EMT's first line of action in caring for a patient having a possible psychiatric emergency is:

   a. restrain the patient at the first sign of aggression.
   b. wait outside for police and other help to arrive.
   c. threaten the patient with restraint to cause him to calm down.
   d. utilize methods of personal interaction.

4. Bystanders at an emergency feel that what is happening is beyond their control and ability to assist and consider the situation to be:

   a. a crisis.
   b. an emotional emergency.
   c. a disaster.
   d. none of the above.

5. Throughout care to a deaf patient, the EMT should:

   a. not waste valuable time trying to explain things, since the patient cannot hear.
   b. pretend to understand unclear responses, so as not to embarrass the patient.
   c. yell in the patient's ear.
   d. maintain face-to-face contact at all times.

6. The restraint and forcible moving of aggressive patients by the EMT in most states is:

   a. allowed if the patient's family requests it.
   b. not permitted unless ordered by a law enforcement official.
   c. provided for in the medical practices act for EMTs.
   d. not allowed under any circumstances.

# SPECIAL PATIENTS AND BEHAVIORAL PROBLEMS

7. When the EMT deals with a blind patient he or she should:
   a. avoid using words like "see" and "look," as these may offend the blind patient.
   b. constantly inform the patient what will be done or touched next.
   c. not assist the patient in moving since blind patients prefer to be independent.
   d. assist the blind patient by walking behind them.

8. The EMT initially restrains a violent patient with police assistance. Later, en route to the hospital, the patient calms down, and asks you to remove the restraints. The EMT should:
   a. remove the restraints if they cause pain.
   b. remove the restraints if the family is riding in the ambulance.
   c. remove the restraints only if the police are present.
   d. not remove restraints until in the hospital.

9. Emotional involvement may cause an EMT to suffer:
   a. burnout.
   b. personal interaction.
   c. lack of reward.
   d. aggressive behavior.

10. A situation in which the patient is not acting as expected is called:
    a. a crisis.
    b. role playing.
    c. personal interaction.
    d. an emotional emergency.

11. The EMT is called to provide care for an attempted suicide. Upon arrival, the patient is found to be in possession of a weapon. The EMT should:
    a. joke with the patient.
    b. withdraw carefully if he or she can.
    c. attempt to seize the weapon.
    d. have the family disarm the patient.

12. During a patient interview, an elderly patient often appears unresponsive to your questions. This may be due to:
    a. distrust of younger people.
    b. fear.
    c. a hearing problem.
    d. pain.

13. A patient characterized by an EMT as having an emotional emergency often:
    a. simply needs more time to cope with the stress of the emergency.
    b. is dangerous to himself or to others.
    c. needs to be restrained.
    d. needs to be pressured into making choices for himself.

14. One of the most crucial things an EMT can do when caring for a crime victim is:
    a. look for evidence.
    b. provide emotional support and reassurance.
    c. question the patient about the crime for the police.
    d. immediately remove the patient from the scene to a less stressful environment.

15. When an EMT is called to transport an aggressive psychiatric patient and the police are not on the scene, the EMT should:
    a. capture and restrain the patient so that he or she can be held until the police arrive.
    b. capture the patient but not restrain him, and wait for the police.
    c. not attempt to capture or restrain the patient until police assistance arrives.
    d. have the family hold down the patient so the EMTs can restrain and treat the patient.

## SITUATIONS FOR FURTHER DISCUSSION

1. You are called to treat a 30-year-old man who appears to be guarding his abdomen. When you attempt to question him, he speaks a foreign language.

   a. What do your primary and secondary surveys indicate the problem to be?

   b. What factors allow you to come to this conclusion?

# SPECIAL PATIENTS AND BEHAVIORAL PROBLEMS 121

c. What factors caused you to rule out other conditions?

d. What is the correct emergency treatment for this patient and in what order?

e. In what position will you transport this patient?

f. What continuing care will you provide for this patient en route to the hospital?

g. What common allied problems might you expect to find or see develop with this patient's condition?

h. What is the urgency of transportation to the hospital for this patient?

i. What would be your radio report to the hospital regarding the situation and present condition of the patient?

2. You are called by family members to treat a 36-year-old male who fell down a flight of stairs after having had a few drinks. He is conscious and refuses your care. The family members demand that you take him to the hospital, and a shouting match develops between the patient and his family. Now as you attempt to explain to the patient why you feel that he should go to hospital, he becomes aggressive.

   a. What do your primary and secondary surveys indicate the problem to be?

   b. What factors allow you to come to this conclusion?

   c. What factors caused you to rule out other conditions?

   d. What is the correct emergency treatment for this patient and in what order?

   e. In what position will you transport this patient?

   f. What continuing care will you provide for this patient en route to the hospital?

**122** SPECIAL PATIENTS AND BEHAVIORAL PROBLEMS

    g. What common allied problems might you expect to find or see develop with this patient's condition?

    h. What is the urgency of transportation to the hospital for this patient?

    i. What would be your radio report to the hospital regarding the situation and present condition of the patient?

**3.** You are called by a man to treat his wife. He suspects that she has taken an overdose of Valium. When you arrive, she is conscious but occasionally groggy. She refuses your assistance.

    a. What do your primary and secondary surveys indicate the problem to be?

    b. What factors allow you to come to this conclusion?

    c. What factors caused you to rule out other conditions?

    d. What is the correct emergency treatment for this patient and in what order?

    e. In what position will you transport this patient?

    f. What continuing care will you provide for this patient en route to the hospital?

    g. What common allied problems might you expect to find or see develop with this patient's condition?

    h. What is the urgency of transportation to the hospital for this patient?

    i. What would be your radio report to the hospital regarding the situation and present condition of the patient?

# 20

# Triage and Disaster Management

- *Multiple Patient Situations*
- *Disasters*

---

1. The term used to describe situations in which there are more than one patient is:

   a. multitrauma.
   b. multicasualty.
   c. disaster.
   d. maxitrauma.

2. In a multivictim triage situation, a patient with minor fractures and stable vital signs should be placed in:

   a. highest priority.
   b. second priority.
   c. delayed priority.
   d. lowest priority.

3. In a disaster situation, a patient is assessed as having a possible spine fracture, with loss of sensation below the waist. Vital signs are stable. This patient is assigned:

   a. highest priority.
   b. second priority.
   c. delayed priority.
   d. lowest priority.

4. A red triage tag indicates:

   a. highest priority.
   b. second priority.
   c. delayed priority.
   d. lowest priority.

5. A decapitation victim in any mass casualty situation would be placed in the:

   a. highest priority.
   b. second priority.
   c. delayed priority.
   d. lowest priority.

6. The process by which the EMT sorts patients into categories of priority for care and transport is called:

   a. sorting.
   b. staging.
   c. tagging.
   d. triage.

7. A young child found in a disaster situation with fractures to the lower leg, upper arm, and wrist would be placed in:

   a. highest priority.
   b. second priority.
   c. delayed priority.
   d. lowest priority.

8. A patient with an evisceration and stable vital signs in a multicasualty situation should be classified as:

   a. highest priority.
   b. second priority.
   c. delayed priority.
   d. lowest priority.

9. At the scene of a mass casualty, the EMT finds an unconscious, elderly patient with no obvious signs of injury. This patient should be classified as:

   a. highest priority.
   b. second priority.
   c. delayed priority.
   d. lowest priority.

10. The driver of a bus that flipped over while carrying a group of children on a field trip is found to have suffered severe burns to his arms and chest while trying to put out a fire in the engine compartment. In which priority should the driver be placed?

    a. Highest priority
    b. Second priority
    c. Delayed priority
    d. Lowest priority

11. Once a disaster victim has been triaged, his priority:

    a. can change only if his condition worsens.
    b. must stay the same until all patients are evaluated.
    c. constantly becomes more urgent over time.
    d. can change depending on the number of patients, other injuries, and available resources.

12. At the scene of a school explosion, a patient is found conscious but suffering a head injury. His priority should be:

    a. highest priority.
    b. second priority.
    c. delayed priority.
    d. lowest priority.

13. The principal of a school that has just collapsed is assisting the triage team in identifying patients, when he suddenly clutches his chest and is in severe pain. He should be classified as:

    a. highest priority.
    b. second priority.
    c. delayed priority.
    d. lowest priority.

14. A victim is found early in the removal process before many EMTs have arrived at the scene of a building collapse involving at least 30 victims. He appears to be in cardiac arrest. The triaging EMT should classify this patient as:

    a. highest priority.
    b. second priority.
    c. delayed priority.
    d. lowest priority.

15. Triage tags should be:

    a. used sparingly.
    b. used even if there are only one or two patients.
    c. large enough for a complete medical history.
    d. brightly colored and able to be filled out quickly.

16. A patient in a mass casualty situation with a pneumothorax should be assigned as:

    a. highest priority.
    b. second priority.
    c. delayed priority.
    d. lowest priority.

17. At the scene of a building collapse, the triage EMT classifies a patient with uncontrollable hemorrhage from the axilla as:

    a. highest priority.
    b. second priority.
    c. delayed priority.
    d. lowest priority.

18. The EMT should classify a patient found in a mass casualty situation suffering from multiple fractures and moderate bleeding in which priority?

    a. Highest priority
    b. Second priority
    c. Delayed priority
    d. Lowest priority

19. When an ambulance arrives at the scene of a multicasualty situation:

    a. EMTs should transport the most seriously injured patients first.
    b. EMTs should transport only one patient per vehicle.
    c. the driver should assist the EMTs with assessment and treatment.
    d. the driver should not leave the vehicle.

20. In a multicasualty triage situation, a patient found with severe head injuries would typically be classified as:

    a. highest priority.
    b. second priority.
    c. delayed priority.
    d. lowest priority.

## SITUATIONS FOR FURTHER DISCUSSION

1. You have been assigned to stabilize three victims who were injured in a building collapse. There are many victims in other parts of the building, and you are told that it may be 20 or 30 minutes before additional rescuers and equipment are available. The first victim is screaming hysterically and complains that she cannot feel her legs. The second victim is moaning, appears cyanotic, and has deformity in the right thigh. The third victim is motionless, silent, and the head appears flexed, possibly occluding the airway.

   a. What do your primary and secondary surveys indicate the problem to be?

   b. What factors allow you to come to this conclusion?

   c. What factors caused you to rule out other conditions?

   d. What is the correct emergency treatment for this patient and in what order?

   e. In what position will you transport this patient?

   f. What continuing care will you provide for this patient en route to the hospital?

   g. What common allied problems might you expect to find or see develop with this patient's condition?

   h. What is the urgency of transportation to the hospital for this patient?

   i. What would be your radio report to the hospital regarding the situation and present condition of the patient?

2. You are responsible for coordinating transport from a multicasualty situation where a bus carrying school children was struck by a train. At this moment, you have only one ambulance available to transport and the following patients: the driver of the bus, who has a flail chest and appears cyanotic; a 12-year-old boy with a spinal injury; a 17-year-old girl with a sucking chest wound who appears cyanotic; three children with assorted bumps and bruises; a 14-year-old girl with a fractured femur who does not appear cyanotic; and an elderly bystander who has gone into cardiac arrest.

   a. What do your primary and secondary surveys indicate the problem to be?

## 126 TRIAGE AND DISASTER MANAGEMENT

b. What factors allow you to come to this conclusion?

c. What factors caused you to rule out other conditions?

d. What is the correct emergency treatment for this patient and in what order?

e. In what position will you transport this patient?

f. What continuing care will you provide for this patient en route to the hospital?

g. What common allied problems might you expect to find or see develop with this patient's condition?

h. What is the urgency of transportation to the hospital for this patient?

i. What would be your radio report to the hospital regarding the situation and present condition of the patient?

3. While assisting at a multicasualty situation, a firefighter develops chest pain and shortness of breath.

a. What do your primary and secondary surveys indicate the problem to be?

b. What factors allow you to come to this conclusion?

c. What factors caused you to rule out other conditions?

d. What is the correct emergency treatment for this patient and in what order?

e. In what position will you transport this patient?

f. What continuing care will you provide for this patient en route to the hospital?

g. What common allied problems might you expect to find or see develop with this patient's condition?

h. What is the urgency of transportation to the hospital for this patient?

i. What would be your radio report to the hospital regarding the situation and present condition of the patient?

4. While triaging at the scene of a school bus accident, the triage leader finds his own child, who has been badly injured.

   a. What do your primary and secondary surveys indicate the problem to be?

   b. What factors allow you to come to this conclusion?

c. What factors caused you to rule out other conditions?

d. What is the correct emergency treatment for this patient and in what order?

e. In what position will you transport this patient?

f. What continuing care will you provide for this patient en route to the hospital?

g. What common allied problems might you expect to find or see develop with this patient's condition?

h. What is the urgency of transportation to the hospital for this patient?

i. What would be your radio report to the hospital regarding the situation and present condition of the patient?

# 21

# Preparing for the Ambulance Run

- *The Ambulance*

---

**SITUATIONS FOR FURTHER DISCUSSION**

1. Obtain a copy of your organization's ambulance inspection sheet and conduct a preshift ambulance inspection of the ambulance's mechanical systems.

2. Obtain a copy of your organization's ambulance equipment/supplies inventory sheet. Locate these items in the ambulance and familiarize yourself with their operation.

# 22

# Responding to the Call for Help

- *Receiving the Call for Help*
- *Driving the Ambulance*
- *Responding to the Scene of a Vehicle Accident*
- *Positioning the Ambulance*

---

1. Studies have shown that the continuous use of the siren:

    a. calms the patient.
    b. gets the patient to the hospital faster and safer.
    c. reassures the patient's family.
    d. increases the driving speed of inexperienced drivers by 10 to 15 mph.

2. The number of feet that a vehicle travels from the time the driver decides to stop until the vehicle actually stops is:

    a. constant regardless of speed.
    b. independent of road conditions.
    c. called stopping distance.
    d. called reaction distance.

3. While driving the ambulance on an emergency run, the driver feels the accelerator stick. The driver should:

    a. shift to neutral, pull over, and stop.
    b. reach down and pull the accelerator up.
    c. jam on the brakes.
    d. turn on the siren.

4. When responding to an accident that involves the leaking of dangerous chemicals, the ambulance driver should park:

    a. about 50 feet away.
    b. downwind.
    c. upwind only if fumes are evident.
    d. upwind at all times.

5. The use of the siren during transport:

    a. gives the ambulance the right of way.
    b. may increase the fear and anxiety of the patient.
    c. calms and reassures the patient.
    d. reassures the family.

6. The distance that the ambulance travels from time the driver decides to stop until the moment his foot applies the brake is called:

    a. stopping distance.
    b. reaction distance.
    c. reaction time.
    d. braking distance.

7. In wet weather, there is a tendency for a film of water to develop between the road and the tires, making steering virtually impossible. This condition:

    a. is called hydroplaning and is corrected by slowing down.
    b. is called hydroplaning and is corrected by speeding up.
    c. is called standing water.
    d. does not affect ambulances because of weight and use of special tires.

8. At the scene of a roadway accident involving high explosives, the ambulance driver should park:

    a. upwind.
    b. downwind.

129

c. 100 feet away upwind.
d. at least 2000 feet away.

9. The most effective warning device for the ambulance driver to use when the ambulance is up close to another vehicle usually is:

   a. the horn.
   b. the siren.
   c. the public address.
   d. the warning lights.

10. When slowing the ambulance on a slippery surface, the driver should:

    a. lock the brakes.
    b. use the parking brake.
    c. use the parking brake and low gear.
    d. pump the brakes.

11. When the ambulance is positioned at a roadway accident where there is no available space off the road to park, the driver should position the ambulance:

    a. between the wreckage and oncoming traffic, about 50 feet away.
    b. between the wreckage and oncoming traffic, but more than 50 feet away.
    c. beyond the wreckage, within 50 feet.
    d. beyond the wreckage, but more than 50 feet away.

12. At the scene of a burning vehicle accident, the ambulance should be positioned:

    a. downwind.
    b. uphill, no closer than 50 feet.
    c. no closer than 50 feet.
    d. upwind, uphill, and more than 100 feet away.

13. The most effective daytime visual warning device is (are) the:

    a. four-way flashers.
    b. headlights.
    c. flashing beacons.
    d. spot light.

14. When the ambulance skids on a slippery surface, the driver should steer:

    a. in the opposite direction of the skid and pump the brakes.
    b. in the opposite direction of the skid and lock the brakes.
    c. in the direction of the skid.
    d. in the direction of the skid and lock the brakes.

15. If the ambulance must be positioned on the roadway facing oncoming traffic at night, the driver should:

    a. turn off the headlights.
    b. turn on the headlights but turn off the flashers.
    c. leave the siren on.
    d. point spot lights directly at oncoming traffic.

16. The ambulance's audible and visual warning devices:

    a. ask the drivers of other vehicles to clear the way for the ambulance.
    b. demand clearance of other vehicles ahead.
    c. physically clear the road.
    d. must be used whenever the ambulance is in operation.

17. After driving the ambulance through standing water, the driver should:

    a. stop until the brakes dry.
    b. tap the brakes lightly several times to dry out the brakes.
    c. continue to drive while holding moderate pressure with the other foot on the brake pedal.
    d. not be concerned, since the brake units are sealed.

18. At accidents involving downed electrical wires and/or damaged utility poles, the danger zone should extend:

    a. five feet in all directions from the end of the wire.
    b. ten feet in all directions from the end of the wire.
    c. one pole length to either side of the downed wire.
    d. beyond each intact pole for a full span and to the sides for the distance that the severed wires can reach.

## SITUATIONS FOR FURTHER DISCUSSION

1. While responding to an accident scene, the most direct route will take you past an elementary school just as school is dismissed.

   a. Describe which of your audible and visual warning devices would be operating.

b. What would be the speed of the vehicle?

c. What special driving techniques (if any) would be necessary in this situation?

d. What would be your report to your dispatcher?

2. While driving the ambulance on an emergency run during a rainstorm, the vehicle begins to hydroplane.

   a. Describe which of your audible and visual warning devices would be operating.

   b. What would be the speed of the vehicle?

   c. What special driving techniques (if any) would be necessary in this situation?

d. What would be your report to your dispatcher?

3. While responding to a sick call during a snowstorm, the ambulance skids off the road.

   a. Describe which of your audible and visual warning devices would be operating.

   b. What would be the speed of the vehicle?

   c. What special driving techniques (if any) would be necessary in this situation?

   d. What would be your report to your dispatcher?

# 23

# Transferring Patients to the Ambulance

- *Basic Principles of Moving Patients*
- *Transferring the Patient*
- *Spine Boards*

---

1. Which type of carrying device requires access to the patient from all sides?

    a. Scoop style stretcher
    b. Stair chair stretcher
    c. Stokes stretcher
    d. Pole stretcher

2. If the EMT must use a stair chair to transport a patient down stairs:

    a. all straps should be loosened temporarily.
    b. the stair chair should be wheeled over each step carefully.
    c. the foot end EMT should face toward the direction of travel.
    d. the foot end EMT should face the patient.

3. Which type of carrying device is not recommended for use with unconscious or disoriented patients?

    a. Stokes stretcher
    b. Scoop style stretcher
    c. Wheeled ambulance stretcher
    d. Stair chair stretcher

4. When placing the patient in a Stokes stretcher, the EMT should:

    a. line the basket with blankets before placing the patient in the basket.
    b. attach all lifting bridles and lines before placing the patient in the basket.
    c. remove the cervical collar.
    d. use the straddle lift technique.

5. When using any of the "one-rescuer drags," the EMT must:

    a. pull in the direction across from the long axis of the body.
    b. pull in the direction of the long axis of the body.
    c. never pull from the feet.
    d. be on his hands and knees.

6. To use a scoop-style stretcher, the EMTs should:

    a. unfasten only the foot end and "scissor" the two halves together.
    b. adjust the length after the patient is on the stretcher.
    c. place both halves of the stretcher under the patient at the same time.
    d. latch the head end first and then secure the foot end latch.

7. If the pathway from the patient to the ambulance involves obstacles and inclines, what is the carrying device of choice?

    a. Stair chair stretcher
    b. Stokes stretcher
    c. Pole stretcher
    d. Wheeled ambulance stretcher

8. The blanket lift for a non-spine-injured patient is best accomplished using:
   a. two rescuers.
   b. three rescuers.
   c. four rescuers.
   d. five rescuers.

9. If an accident victim is found lying between the front seat and dashboard, the EMT should:
   a. slide the patient onto a long board held at the edge of the door opening.
   b. displace the front seat and both doors.
   c. remove the roof.
   d. move the patient to a sitting position so a short spine board can be applied.

10. The EMTs should load the wheeled ambulance stretcher into the ambulance using the:
    a. end carry.
    b. side carry.
    c. cradle carry.
    d. fireman's carry.

11. To transfer a sitting patient to a stair chair using a modified direct carry, the foot-end EMT should place his or her arms under the:
    a. thighs and at midcalf.
    b. small of the back.
    c. small of the back and thighs.
    d. small of the back and at midcalf.

12. Which of the following is considered safest for placing a supine, spine-injured patient onto a long spine board?
    a. Scoop style stretcher
    b. Log roll
    c. Four-rescuer straddle
    d. Rope sling

13. The EMT should secure a conscious patient to a stair chair using:
    a. a blanket secured to the device at the shoulders.
    b. three straps at the chest, waist, and legs.
    c. two straps at the chest and waist.
    d. one strap at the waist.

14. The most common technique for transferring a patient from a bed to the wheeled ambulance stretcher is the:
    a. direct carry method.
    b. draw sheet method.
    c. blanket lift method.
    d. straddle slide method.

## SITUATIONS FOR FURTHER DISCUSSION

1. A spine-injured patient must be transported from the third floor of an apartment building to the street level. There is no elevator in the building.

   a. How will you place the patient onto the carrying device you have chosen?

   b. Which device will you use to transfer this patient?

   c. What factors caused you to rule out other devices?

   d. What is the correct strapping sequence for this device and patient and in what order?

   e. In what position will you transport this patient?

   f. How many trained responders are required to carry this patient on this device?

   g. Where would you place the EMTs to carry this patient?

**134** TRANSFERRING PATIENTS TO THE AMBULANCE

2. A patient with a fractured femur must be carried from the basement to the first floor.

   a. How will you place the patient onto the carrying device you have chosen?

   b. Which device will you use to transfer this patient?

   c. What factors caused you to rule out other devices?

   d. What is the correct strapping sequence for this device and patient and in what order?

   e. In what position will you transport this patient?

   f. How many trained responders are required to carry this patient on this device?

   g. Where would you place the EMTs to carry this patient?

3. A spine-injured patient must be placed on a long spine board. Assume that the patient is found in the supine position.

   a. How will you place the patient onto the carrying device you have chosen?

   b. Which device will you use to transfer this patient?

   c. What factors caused you to rule out other devices?

   d. What is the correct strapping sequence for this device and patient and in what order?

   e. In what position will you transport this patient?

   f. How many trained responders are required to carry this patient on this device?

   g. Where would you place the EMTs to carry this patient?

## TRANSFERRING PATIENTS TO THE AMBULANCE 135

4. A non-spine-injured patient must be removed quickly from a building due to a fire. Assume that you are alone with the patient.

   a. How will you place the patient onto the carrying device you have chosen?

   b. Which device will you use to transfer this patient?

   c. What factors caused you to rule out other devices?

   d. What is the correct strapping sequence for this device and patient and in what order?

   e. In what position will you transport this patient?

   f. How many trained responders are required to carry this patient on this device?

   g. Where would you place the EMTs to carry this patient?

5. A possible spine-injured patient must be removed from a burning building. Assume that you are alone in this situation.

   a. How will you place the patient onto the carrying device you have chosen?

   b. Which device will you use to transfer this patient?

   c. What factors caused you to rule out other devices?

   d. What is the correct strapping sequence for this device and patient and in what order?

   e. In what position will you transport this patient?

   f. How many trained responders are required to carry this patient on this device?

   g. Where would you place the EMTs to carry this patient?

**136** TRANSFERRING PATIENTS TO THE AMBULANCE

6. A non-spine-injured patient must be placed on the wheeled ambulance cot. Assume that two EMTs are present.

   a. How will you place the patient onto the carrying device you have chosen?

   b. Which device will you use to transfer this patient?

   c. What factors caused you to rule out other devices?

   d. What is the correct strapping sequence for this device and patient and in what order?

   e. In what position will you transport this patient?

   f. How many trained responders are required to carry this patient on this device?

   g. Where would you place the EMTs to carry this patient?

7. You must remove a spine-injured patient from a sports car with bucket seats.

   a. How will you place the patient onto the carrying device you have chosen?

   b. Which device will you use to transfer this patient?

   c. What factors caused you to rule out other devices?

   d. What is the correct strapping sequence for this device and patient and in what order?

   e. In what position will you transport this patient?

   f. How many trained responders are required to carry this patient on this device?

   g. Where would you place the EMTs to carry this patient?

TRANSFERRING PATIENTS TO THE AMBULANCE   137

8. You must remove a spine-injured patient from the rear floor of a two-door vehicle.

   a. How will you place the patient onto the carrying device you have chosen?

   b. Which device will you use to transfer this patient?

   c. What factors caused you to rule out other devices?

   d. What is the correct strapping sequence for this device and patient and in what order?

   e. In what position will you transport this patient?

   f. How many trained responders are required to carry this patient on this device?

   g. Where would you place the EMTs to carry this patient?

9. You must remove a patient with a fractured femur from the driver's seat of a two-door vehicle.

   a. How will you place the patient onto the carrying device you have chosen?

   b. Which device will you use to transfer this patient?

   c. What factors caused you to rule out other devices?

   d. What is the correct strapping sequence for this device and patient and in what order?

   e. In what position will you transport this patient?

   f. How many trained responders are required to carry this patient on this device?

   g. Where would you place the EMTs to carry this patient?

# 24

# Transporting the Patient to a Hospital

- *Preparing the Patient for Transport*
- *Caring for the Patient While En Route to the Hospital*
- *Radio Communications During Transport*
- *Transferring the Patient to the Care of the Emergency Department Personnel*

---

1. Prior to closing the rear doors of the ambulance, the EMT must:
   a. be sure that the emergency flashers are operating correctly.
   b. make sure the ambulance stretcher is securely in place.
   c. have notified the hospital of the patient and his or her condition.
   d. open a window for ventilation.

2. When a patient who has been bandaged at the scene is transported, the EMT must:
   a. soak the dressings with normal saline while en route to the hospital.
   b. replace the dressings and bandages with new sterile dressings since the ambulance compartment is a cleaner environment than the scene.
   c. remove the dressings and spray the injury site with an antibiotic.
   d. keep the bandaged areas uncovered from blankets or sheets or he or she may observe the areas for resumed hemorrhage.

3. Occasionally, while moving the patient on the wheeled ambulance stretcher, it may be necessary to:
   a. secure the patient in a supine position for a short period of time to maintain balance over rough terrain; once in the ambulance, the patient may be placed in the proper position for his or her condition.
   b. remove the securing straps if they pull at the patient while transporting the stretcher down a short flight of stairs.
   c. roll the stretcher in the elevated position over rough terrain such as a lawn.
   d. roll the stretcher sideways in the elevated position.

4. When transporting a patient whose injuries have required splinting, the EMT should:
   a. not secure the patient to the stretcher with straps.
   b. check air splints for proper pressure again in the ambulance.
   c. apply more traction to all splinted femur fractures.
   d. remove all splints during transportation to improve circulation.

5. Smoking is allowed in the ambulance:
   a. only when there is not a patient being transported.
   b. only when oxygen is not in use.

c. only by family members in the driver's compartment.
   d. at no time and under no circumstances.

6. When transporting a patient with a known heart or respiratory condition who may suffer cardiac arrest, the EMT should:
   a. place a short board under the patient prior to transport, even if this may be uncomfortable.
   b. have a family member ride with the patient in the patient compartment.
   c. call the hospital and ask for instructions.
   d. not transport, and await the arrival of a paramedic unit to do the transport.

7. The hysterical 58-year-old wife of a heart attack patient should:
   a. ride in the patient compartment.
   b. ride in the driver's compartment.
   c. be sent to the hospital in a police cruiser.
   d. be left at home alone to minimize aggravation to the patient.

8. Security straps applied to secure the patient during removal from the scene to the ambulance should:
   a. be removed when at the bottom of the stairs.
   b. be adjusted when the patient reaches the ambulance.
   c. be tightened when the patient reaches the ambulance.
   d. be loosened when the patient reaches the ambulance.

9. Once the wheeled ambulance stretcher is lifted into the ambulance, the EMTs must be certain that:
   a. the forward catch is engaged.
   b. the rear catch is locked.
   c. both the forward and rear catches are engaged and locked.
   d. all straps and blankets are removed so the patient may be observed during transportation.

### SITUATIONS FOR FURTHER DISCUSSIONS

1. Using two EMTs, place a patient on a wheeled ambulance cot inside the ambulance and prepare for transport.
   a. Describe the status of the lights and siren during transport of this patient.
   b. What continuing care will you provide for this patient en route to the hospital?
   c. What common allied problems might you expect to find or see develop with this patient's condition?
   d. What is the urgency of transportation to the hospital for this patient?
   e. What would be your radio report to the hospital regarding the situation and present condition of the patient?

2. Using two EMTs, place a patient on a wheeled ambulance cot inside the ambulance while the ambulance is parked with both right wheels off the shoulder and lower than those on the driver's side.
   a. Describe the status of the lights and siren during transport of this patient.
   b. What continuing care will you provide for this patient en route to the hospital?

# 140 TRANSPORTING THE PATIENT TO A HOSPITAL

c. What common allied problems might you expect to find or see develop with this patient's condition?

d. What is the urgency of transportation to the hospital for this patient?

e. What would be your radio report to the hospital regarding the situation and present condition of the patient?

3. A 50-year-old cardiac patient goes into cardiac arrest during transport.

   a. If the situation occurs during the ride to the hospital, is it necessary to stop the ambulance?

   b. Would the driver of the ambulance need to change his speed if this situation occurs during the ride to the hospital?

   c. Describe the status of the lights and siren during transport of this patient.

d. What continuing care will you provide for this patient en route to the hospital?

e. What common allied problems might you expect to find or see develop with this patient's condition?

f. What is the urgency of transportation to the hospital for this patient?

g. What would be your radio report to the hospital regarding the situation and present condition of the patient?

4. While transporting a maternity patient, the baby begins to deliver.

   a. If the situation occurs during the ride to the hospital, is it necessary to stop the ambulance?

   b. Woud the driver of the ambulance need to change his speed if this situation occurs during the ride to the hospital?

## TRANSPORTING THE PATIENT TO A HOSPITAL 141

c. Describe the status of the lights and siren during transport of this patient.

d. What continuing care will you provide for this patient en route to the hospital?

e. What common allied problems might you expect to find or see develop with this patient's condition?

f. What is the urgency of transportation to the hospital for this patient?

g. What would be your radio report to the hospital regarding the situation and present condition of the patient?

5. You are transporting a patient with several severe injuries that were not treated prior to transport at the scene because of low blood pressure and an advanced state of shock. The patient has been placed on a spine board, but no immobilization has been performed. Injuries in addition to suspected spine injury include a fractured femur and a sucking chest wound.

   a. If the situation occurs during the ride to the hospital, is it necessary to stop the ambulance?

   b. Would the driver of the ambulance need to change his speed if this situation occurs during the ride to the hospital?

   c. Describe the status of the lights and siren during transport of this patient?

   d. What continuing care will you provide for this patient en route to the hospital?

   e. What common allied problems might you expect to find or see develop with this patient's condition?

## 142 TRANSPORTING THE PATIENT TO A HOSPITAL

f. What is the urgency of transportation to the hospital for this patient?

g. What would be your radio report to the hospital regarding the situation and present condition of the patient?

# 25

# Terminating the Run

- *Actions That Can Be Taken at the Hospital*
- *Actions That Can Be Taken While En Route to Quarters*
- *Actions That Can Be Taken When in Quarters*

---

**SITUATIONS FOR FURTHER DISCUSSION**

1. Review your organization's equipment exchange policy with your local receiving hospitals.

2. Review your organization's procedures for cleaning and disinfecting nondisposable respiratory equipment.

# 26

# Communications and Reports

- *Communication*
- *Radio Communications*
- *Reports*

---

1. The EMT should use codes when talking to the hospital over the radio:

   a. if the patient can hear the EMT.
   b. if the family is present and can hear the EMT.
   c. if the hospital routinely uses and understands the same codes.
   d. at all times.

2. To transmit a radio message, the EMT should:

   a. speak softly into the microphone.
   b. speak in a normal voice into the microphone.
   c. speak loudly into the microphone.
   d. depress the microphone transmit button for 5 seconds to break other transmissions.

3. The "10-Code," which in most systems indicates "affirmative," is:

   a. 10-0.
   b. 10-1.
   c. 10-4.
   d. 10-10.

4. When using the radio, the EMT should:

   a. always be polite, using "please," "thank you," and other such terms.
   b. ask for a repeat if he or she does not understand part of the message.
   c. talk quickly to free the channel.
   d. give the patient's name over the air so the hospital may check past medical reports.

5. The EMT's written reports:

   a. should be completed as soon as possible.
   b. need not be completed if the patient refused treatment.
   c. should be completed at the end of the shift.
   d. should be completed by the dispatcher.

### SITUATIONS FOR FURTHER DISCUSSION

1. Obtain a copy of the standard "run form" or "incident report" that is used by your service and complete it by using the information in the situations from previous chapters.

2. Write up a radio message as you would transmit it to the hospital to describe the condition of each patient from the situations in previous chapters.

# 27

# Vehicle Rescue

## SECTION ONE: EQUIPMENT FOR VEHICLE RESCUE

- *Supplies and Equipment*
- *Storing Equipment on the Ambulance*

---

**SITUATIONS FOR FURTHER DISCUSSION**

1. Identify the twelve phases of a vehicle rescue operation.

2. Identify your organization's exact role in each of the twelve phases of a vehicle rescue operation.

3. Locate and identify all tools and equipment carried on your vehicle.

# 27

# Vehicle Rescue

## SECTION TWO: MANAGING ACCIDENT-RELATED HAZARDS

- *Hazards*
- *Controlling the Movements of Vehicles*
- *Controlling the Movements of Spectators*
- *Coping with Electrical Hazards*
- *Extinguishing Fires in Accident Vehicles*
- *Coping with Spilled Fuel*
- *Stabilizing Unsteady Vehicles*

---

1. The distance of the farthest warning light device at the scene of a road accident should be:

    a. 50 feet away from the accident.
    b. 100 feet away from the accident.
    c. the stopping distance for the posted speed plus the speed limit in feet from the accident.
    d. the stopping distance for the posted speed from the accident.

2. To warn oncoming drivers of an accident ahead, the EMT should place flares and other warning devices every:

    a. 10 feet.
    b. 25 feet.
    c. 50 feet.
    d. 100 feet.

3. You are called to an accident where electrical wires are down on one of the vehicles. The street lights and lights of nearby houses are dark. You should:

    a. move the wire yourself using a tree limb.
    b. quickly move the patients from danger while the power is off.
    c. do not touch the vehicle or wire until the power company or a trained responder have declared the area safe.
    d. remove the wire yourself while wearing firefighter's gloves and boots for added protection.

4. The battery of a vehicle involved in an accident should be disconnected by:

    a. removing the positive cable first.
    b. removing the negative cable first.
    c. draining the fluid from the battery.
    d. grounding the battery to itself by connecting the negative cable to the positive battery post.

5. In a motor vehicle accident where the vehicle is found on its side, the EMT should:

   a. remove all patients quickly before the vehicle shifts.
   b. stabilize the vehicle with cribbing, wedges, and lines before anyone enters the vehicle.
   c. get bystanders to assist in lowering the vehicle to an upright position.
   d. have bystanders push against the underside of the vehicle as EMTs work inside to remove the patients.

## SITUATIONS FOR FURTHER DISCUSSION

1. While returning from a call, a car in front of you goes off the road and hits a tree. The driver is slumped over the wheel and appears unconscious. The windshield is broken directly over the driver's head. Just as you reach the patient, you smell gas and see smoke coming from under the hood.

   a. What equipment will you need?

   b. What is the minimum number of trained responders needed to gain access to this patient?

   c. What must you do to protect this patient?

   d. What must you do to protect the EMTs?

   e. How will you gain access to this patient?

2. You arrive at an accident scene before fire or rescue personnel. There are victims trapped inside the car, but there is a wire from a utility pole lying across the hood.

   a. What equipment will you need?

   b. What is the minimum number of trained responders needed to gain access to this patient?

   c. What must you do to protect this patient?

   d. What must you do to protect the EMTs?

   e. How will you gain access to this patient?

# 27

# *Vehicle Rescue*

## SECTION THREE: GAINING ACCESS TO VEHICLE OCCUPANTS

- *Gaining Access*
- *Gaining Access Through Door Openings*
- *Entering a Vehicle Through Window Openings*
- *Gaining Access to Injured Occupants by Removing the Roof of an Accident Vehicle*

---

1. Tempered glass is best broken by striking the glass with a:
   a. blunt tool in the center.
   b. blunt tool in the lower corner.
   c. sharp tool in the center.
   d. sharp tool in the lower corner.

2. The preferred order of access routes to trapped vehicle accident victims generally is:
   a. doors, side and rear windows, windshield, roof, and floor.
   b. doors, windshield, side and rear windows, roof, and floor.
   c. side and rear windows, windshield, doors, roof, and floor.
   d. side and rear windows, doors, windshield, roof, and floor.

3. Laminated glass usually is found in:
   a. windshields.
   b. side windows.
   c. rear windows.
   d. mirrors.

4. When tempered glass is broken, it tends to:
   a. form shards.
   b. crack, yet remain intact.
   c. break into many small pieces.
   d. Tempered glass does not break.

### SITUATIONS FOR FURTHER DISCUSSION

1. You are the first unit to arrive at an automobile accident. The vehicle's doors are all jammed, the windows are all rolled up, and the victim appears slumped over the wheel with his head flexed forward.

   a. What equipment will you need?

b. What is the minimum number of trained responders needed to gain access to this patient?

c. What must you do to protect this patient?

d. What must you do to protect the EMTs?

e. How will you gain access to this patient?

# 27

# *Vehicle Rescue*

## SECTION FOUR: DISENTANGLING TRAPPED PERSONS

- *Disentanglement*
- *Protecting the Occupants*
- *Creating Openings in the Wreckage*
- *Removing Mechanisms of Entrapment from Around Victims*

---

1. Which of the following is considered to be a part of disentanglement?

   a. Making a pathway through the wreckage
   b. Immobilization of spinal injuries
   c. Application of spine boards
   d. Removal of the packaged patient from the wreckage

2. Before attempting to cut away a steering wheel, the rescuer should:

   a. remove the windshield.
   b. attempt to move the seat back manually.
   c. remove the roof.
   d. remove the door nearest the patient.

3. The EMT may easily free the victim's feet if they are pinned under the brake or clutch pedals by:

   a. using a hand-operated winch between the steering wheel and the pedal.
   b. using a bumper jack.
   c. using a rope tied to the pedal and the door on the opposite side of the vehicle.
   d. removing the pin from the pedal's hinge point.

4. Before attempting to displace the steering column, the EMT must first:

   a. remove the windshield.
   b. remove the roof.
   c. cut away the steering wheel.
   d. remove the dashboard to create space in which to work.

5. The cutting sequence to remove a car's roof is:

   a. C post, B post, and last A post.
   b. A post, B post, and last C post.
   c. A post and C post.
   d. A post, B post (if any), and notch roof in front of the C post.

6. The EMT must always summon assistance from a rescue squad if disentanglement.

   a. is anticipated, regardless of how simple.
   b. is expected to take more than 10 minutes.
   c. has taken the EMT more than 15 minutes.
   d. involves more than one victim.

150

7. When using a hand winch to widen a door opening, the fixed hook of the winch should be attached to:
   a. the bumper.
   b. a chain attached to a secure point on the frame.
   c. a chain around the door to be pulled.
   d. the door handle of the door to be pulled.

8. Vehicle roof removal by the EMT is made easier by:
   a. cutting the C posts.
   b. dimpling the roof with someone's foot at the hinge point as the roof is folded back.
   c. cutting all of the roof support posts and lifting the roof as a unit.
   d. cutting the roof support posts on the side nearest the victim and bending the roof away from the victim.

9. To obtain the best angle for displacing the steering column using a hand winch and chain, the EMT should:
   a. place the winch on the roof so the pull is straight up.
   b. secure the winch to the opposite side door post.
   c. place cribbing between the cable and dash and secure the winch to the frame under the bumper.
   d. wrap the cable around the lower ring of the steering wheel.

### SITUATIONS FOR FURTHER DISCUSSION

1. While preparing a spine-injured patient for removal from an automobile, it is decided that the door will not open wide enough and the steering wheel will most likely be in the way as you remove the spine-boarded patient.

   a. What equipment will you need?

   b. What is the minimum number of trained responders needed to disentangle this patient?

   c. What must you do to protect this patient?

   d. What must you do to protect the EMTs?

   e. How will you disentangle this patient?

2. While removing a spine-injured patient from an automobile, you find that his left foot is pinned under the brake pedal and cannot be freed.

   a. What equipment will you need?

   b. What is the minimum number of trained responders needed to disentangle this patient?

   c. What must you do to protect this patient?

   d. What must you do to protect the EMTs?

   e. How will you disentangle this patient?

**152** VEHICLE RESCUE SECTION FOUR

3. You arrive at the scene of an automobile accident and find that the driver was not wearing a seat belt and has hit the windshield. He is found with his head protruding through a hole in the windshield.

   a. What equipment will you need?

   b. What is the minimum number of trained responders needed to disentangle this patient?

   c. What must you do to protect this patient?

   d. What must you do to protect the EMTs?

   e. How will you disentangle this patient?

# 28

# Sample Final Examination

1. The sacs located in the lungs, where the exchange of oxygen and carbon dioxide takes place, are called:

   a. lungs.
   b. alveoli.
   c. bronchi.
   d. pleural space.

2. The aorta is the largest:

   a. artery.
   b. auricle.
   c. ventricle.
   d. vein.

3. The stomach:

   a. is a hollow organ in the upper left abdomen.
   b. lies in the pelvic cavity.
   c. stores and concentrates bile.
   d. is a solid organ in the lower abdomen.

4. What is the anatomical term used to describe the section of the spine in the lower back?

   a. Cervical vertebrae
   b. Thoracic vertebrae
   c. Lumbar vertebrae
   d. Sacral vertebrae

5. Which of the following organs is located in all four of the abdominal quadrants?

   a. Liver
   b. Stomach
   c. Large intestine
   d. Bladder

6. How much blood does an average-size male have in his body?

   a. 6 pints
   b. 6 liters
   c. 5 pints
   d. 5 liters

   *5 liters*

7. What percentage of oxygen should an EMT deliver to a patient suffering from emphysema?

   a. 2 percent
   b. 10 percent
   c. 24 percent
   d. 100 percent

   *24%*
   *Mod distress NRM*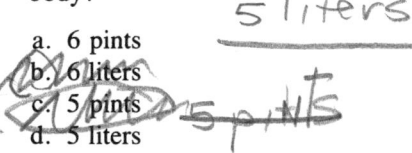

8. An "E" size oxygen tank with a starting pressure of 1800 psi may safely be used at a flow rate of 10 LPM for how long?

   a. 15 minutes
   b. 30 minutes
   c. 45 minutes
   d. 60 minutes

9. Cyanosis in dark-skinned patients can be determined by checking the:

   a. sclera of the eyes.
   b. tongue and lips.
   c. palms.
   d. eyes and earlobes.

   *Lips, tongue*

10. If the EMT's efforts to perform rescue breathing do not result in chest rise, the EMT should:

    a. reposition the head.
    b. administer back blows.
    c. perform abdominal thrusts.
    d. sweep out the mouth using two fingers.

153

11. Which disorder is characterized by normal breathing interrupted by spasms, constrictions, and congestion of the tubes carrying air to the lungs?

    a. Emphysema  *constriction*
    b. Traumatic emphysema
    c. Asthma  *wheezing*  ← circled
    d. Rales  *crackles*

12. If the tongue is obstructing the airway in a patient with a suspected cervical injury, how should the EMT open the airway?

    a. Tilt the patient forward so that the tongue will move.
    b. Move the tongue forward with the fingers.
    c. Hyperextend the head.
    d. Move the mandible forward.  ← circled

13. A partial obstruction of the airway by the tongue is characterized by:

    a. snoring.  ← circled
    b. gurgling.
    c. crowing.
    d. gasping.

14. Gastric distention can be minimized by:

    a. ventilating at a slower rate, but with the same volume of air.
    b. pressing hard to seal the mouth better.
    c. decreasing the pinch to the nose to allow some air to escape.
    d. properly opening the airway and ventilating only until the chest rises normally.  ← circled

15. To perform mouth-to-mouth resuscitation on an infant:

    a. follow the same procedure as for an adult.
    b. blow gentle breaths of air from the cheeks, 20 times per minute, with the head hyperextended.
    c. blow gentle breaths of air from the cheeks, 20 times per minute, with the head in a neutral position.  ← marked
    d. follow the same procedure as for an adult, except ventilate 20 times per minute.

16. The proper-sized oropharyngeal airway can be determined by:  ← circled

    a. measuring from the center of the mouth to the angle of the lower jaw.  ← circled
    b. inserting successive sizes until the patient gags.
    c. measuring from the nose to the chin.
    d. using the largest size that will fit inside the patient's mouth.

17. The proper depth of compressions when providing CPR to an infant is:

    a. ½ to 1 inch.  ← circled
    b. ½ to ¾ inch.
    c. ¼ to ¾ inch.
    d. ¼ to ½ inch.

18. What is the proper ratio of breaths to compressions during one-rescuer CPR to an adult?

    a. 1 to 5
    b. 2 to 5
    c. 2 to 15  ← circled
    d. 1 to 15

19. During a one-minute period of one-rescuer CPR to an adult, the total number of compressions delivered should be:

    a. 60.  ← circled      152
    b. 80.                  152
    c. 90.                  152
    d. 100.                 152

20. What are the signs and symptoms of cardiac arrest?

    a. Weak carotid pulse, constricted pupils, no respirations.
    b. Weak carotid pulse, dilated pupils, no respirations.
    c. Absent carotid pulse, constricted pupils, shallow respirations.
    d. Absent carotid pulse, dilated pupils, no respirations.  ← circled

21. A patient who was breathing at the time of cardiac arrest usually will go into respiratory arrest:

    a. immediately.  ← circled
    b. within 15 seconds before cardiac arrest.
    c. within 30 seconds after cardiac arrest.
    d. 4 to 6 minutes after cardiac arrest.

22. If a carotid pulse cannot be palpated during the five-second pulse check, the EMT should:

    a. reposition the head.
    b. deliver 2 quick breaths.
    c. begin CPR.  ← circled
    d. check the radial pulse for another 5 seconds.

23. Where on the sternum should the heel of the lower hand be placed to deliver cardiac compressions?

    a. The midline
    b. One finger width above the xiphoid process  ← marked
    c. Two finger widths above the xiphoid process
    d. Three finger widths above the substernal notch

24. When during the compression cycle should the rescuer giving ventilations deliver the breath during two-rescuer CPR?

    a. During the 5th downstroke
    b. During the 5th upstroke
    c. During the 15th downstroke
    d. Whenever possible

25. Which of the following is the best indication to let the rescuer know that chest compressions are providing adequate blood flow?

    a. Change in patient's color
    b. Pupils constrict
    c. A second rescuer detects a carotid pulse with each compression.
    d. There is no way to determine this without special instruments.

26. When a rescuer is alone with a cardiac arrest victim and there is no probability of help arriving, he or she should:

    a. telephone for help before starting CPR.
    b. do nothing and wait for help to arrive.
    c. open the patient's airway and then telephone for help.
    d. perform CPR for one minute and then telephone for help.

27. When treating a shock patient without injuries contraindicating elevation of the lower extremities, the patient should be placed:

    a. on a long spine board with the foot end elevated at least 8 inches.
    b. on a long spine board with the foot end elevated between 12 and 18 inches.
    c. lying on a flat surface with the legs inclined from the hips to an elevation at the feet of 12 to 18 inches.
    d. on his or her side on a long spine board with the foot end elevated at least 12 to 18 inches.

28. What type of shock results from the loss of plasma caused by severe burns?
    a. Hypovolemic
    b. Cardiogenic
    c. Septic
    d. Metabolic

29. A conscious patient in shock asks for something to drink. The EMT should give the patient:

    a. anything he or she wants.
    b. coffee or tea.
    c. clear liquids only.
    d. nothing by mouth.

30. Which type of shock is usually considered to be self-correcting?

    a. Cardiogenic
    b. Hemorrhagic
    c. Psychogenic
    d. Respiratory

31. Once applied, a tourniquet:

    a. should be loosened every 10 minutes.
    b. should be loosened every 20 minutes.
    c. should be loosened every 30 minutes.
    d. should not be loosened.

32. A 10-year-old child at a baseball game has a flushed and slightly swollen face and complains of a throbbing headache and tightness in his chest. The EMT should suspect:

    a. asthma.
    b. concussion.
    c. epilepsy.
    d. anaphylaxsis.

33. When a patient appears to be bleeding internally, the EMT should:

    a. rush the patient to the hospital.
    b. keep the patient comfortable.
    c. apply as much pressure as possible over the bleeding area.
    d. administer oxygen, treat for shock, and transport.

34. Bleeding from large veins from the neck should be considered serious because:

    a. the veins are close to the brain.
    b. venous bleeding will cause an immediate reduction in oxygen supply to the brain.
    c. it is difficult to maintain direct pressure to the neck without endangering the airway.
    d. there is a possibility that air will enter the wound and travel to the heart.

35. The EMT can control severe hemorrhage from the forearm by applying pressure over the:

    a. radial artery.
    b. brachial artery.
    c. subclavian artery.
    d. temporal artery.

36. Which of the following symptoms indicate a patient in shock?

    a. Slow, strong pulse; dizziness; nausea; cold perspiration
    b. Blank expression; cold extremities; regular breathing
    c. Rapid, weak pulse; irregular breathing; clammy skin
    d. Blank expression; chills; dry skin; unconsciousness

37. The open wound characterized by jagged skin edges and free bleeding is called a(n):

    a. abrasion.
    b. incision.
    c. laceration.
    d. puncture.

38. When bandaging the extremities, the EMT should:

    a. apply bandages tightly over the fingers and toes.
    b. apply bandages loosely over the fingers and toes.
    c. leave the fingers or toes exposed whenever possible.
    d. apply bandages over the fingers and toes only during cold weather.

39. An impaled object should be removed only if it is in the:

    a. abdomen.
    b. cheek.
    c. chest.
    d. skull.

40. If an area of skin such as a portion of the ear is completely avulsed, it should be:

    a. held in place on the injury site with tape.
    b. discarded, since it is now dead tissue.
    c. placed in a container of sterile saline and transported with the patient.
    d. wrapped in a sterile dressing and kept as cool as possible.

41. In what position should a sucking chest wound patient be transported?

    a. Lying on the injured side
    b. Lying on the uninjured side
    c. Semireclining
    d. Supine

42. In a patient with a flail chest, the loose chest segment will:

    a. move in and out with the rest of the chest.
    b. move in the opposite direction from the rest of the chest.
    c. remain stationary as the chest moves in and out.
    d. change size as the chest moves in and out.

43. The EMT should treat a lacerated globe of the eye by:

    a. applying direct pressure.
    b. covering with a loose dressing.
    c. applying a pressure dressing.
    d. leaving it uncovered so blood may flow unrestricted.

44. The female genitalia are:

    a. located in the abdominal cavity.
    b. exterior to the body.
    c. located in the pelvic cavity.
    d. located in the thoracic cavity.

45. In treating a patient with abdominal injuries, the EMT should transport the patient on his or her:

    a. back with legs flexed.
    b. side with head up.
    c. side with head down.
    d. stomach with head flexed.

46. If a patient is found with an impaled object in the abdomen, the EMT should:

    a. remove it if the patient shows signs of shock.
    b. remove it if internal organs are protruding.
    c. not remove it unless patient is thrashing about.
    d. not remove it under any circumstances.

47. Which of the following devices is the emergency treatment of choice for immobilizing a fractured femur?

    a. Air splint
    b. Traction splint
    c. Ladder splint
    d. Padded long splint

48. A fracture of the elbow should always be immobilized:

    a. in a fully extended, straight position.
    b. in a bent position.
    c. after the victim has been secured to a back board.
    d. in the position in which it is found.

49. How can the EMT determine whether an air splint is properly inflated?

   a. Condensation appears inside the splint.
   b. The exposed fingers or toes become red.
   c. The victim feels pressure along the axis of the fracture.
   d. The splint can be dented with moderate pressure.

50. After splinting a fractured elbow, the radial pulse in the injured arm is very weak and the patient complains of loss of sensation. The EMT should:

   a. loosen the bandages securing the splint.
   b. transport the patient immediately.
   c. unsplint the arm, reposition it, and then resplint it again.
   d. position the splinted arm lower than the rest of the body to improve circulation.

51. A traction splint is best indicated to stabilize a fracture of the:

   a. tibia.
   b. femur.
   c. humerus.
   d. fibula.

52. When splinting a fractured femur, the EMT should apply mechanical traction until:

   a. manual traction is replaced.
   b. the fracture is reduced.
   c. the bone ends slip together.
   d. 30 pounds of countertraction are applied.

53. The grating noise heard when a fractured limb is moved is called

   a. Synovial noise
   b. Crepitus
   c. Articulation
   d. Periosteum

54. At the scene of an automobile accident, a victim has clear, waterlike fluid seeping from his ears. You should:

   a. loosely cover the ears with a sterile dressing.
   b. do nothing, since this is a normal finding in a head injury.
   c. collect the fluid in a sterile container for later analysis.
   d. pack the ears with sterile dressings to prevent further fluid loss.

55. Which of the following conditions is characterized by unequal size of the pupils?

   a. Hemorrhagic shock
   b. Loss of consciousness
   c. Head injury
   d. Use of narcotics

56. Injury to what section of the vertebral column may result in immediate death?

   a. Cervical
   b. Thoracic
   c. Lumbar
   d. Coccygeal

57. What does bleeding from the ears and discoloration of the soft tissues under the eyes in an unconscious accident victim indicate?

   a. Stroke
   b. Concussion
   c. Fractured skull
   d. Cerebral thrombosis

58. A patient with a head injury has the following vitals: blood pressure 80 systolic, and respirations 20 and shallow. The EMT should treat this patient by placing the patient:

   a. with the head slightly elevated.
   b. in the shock position.
   c. in the Trendelenburg position.
   d. on his or her side with the head elevated.

59. While treating a head-injury patient, the patient goes into shock. The EMT should look for:

   a. concussion.
   b. cerebral edema.
   c. epidural hematoma.
   d. another serious injury.

60. To treat a bleeding, open head wound, the EMT should:

   a. apply a snug pressure bandage to control bleeding.
   b. apply a loose sterile dressing to aid the clotting process.
   c. apply pressure to the carotid artery.
   d. elevate the patient's head and apply firm pressure.

61. When immobilizing a spine-injured patient to a long spineboard, manual hand stabilization must be maintained until:

    a. a soft cervical collar is applied.
    b. a rigid cervical collar is applied.
    c. the head is secured to the long spine board.
    d. the patient is completely secured to the long spine board.

62. If a suspected spine-injured patient must be moved, the spinal cord should be kept:

    a. well padded.
    b. in traction.
    c. tightly wrapped.
    d. in a straight line.

63. Which technique is the preferred method to place a suspected spine-injured patient onto a long spine board?

    a. Log roll
    b. Blanket lift
    c. Four-man straddle slide
    d. Split litter

64. Priapism is considered to be a reliable sign of:

    a. spinal injury.
    b. abdominal injury.
    c. chest injury.
    d. shock.

65. The first step in immobilizing an unconscious accident patient to a short spine board is:

    a. apply a cervical collar.
    b. position the board behind the patient.
    c. maintain manual stabilization on the patient's head.
    d. immobilize extremity fractures.

66. When the convulsive seizure of an epileptic has stopped, the patient will probably be:

    a. excited and restless.
    b. very hungry and thirsty.
    c. drowsy and need sleep.
    d. perfectly normal.

67. A child has been playing in the cellar, where he found and drank fluid from an unmarked container. When you arrive, the child is coughing and gagging. The child's mouth and lips appear to be burned. You should:

    a. induce vomiting.
    b. dilute and administer syrup of ipecac.
    c. call poison control.
    d. dilute using water.

68. Which of the following is considered a true emergency requiring immediate transportation to the hospital?

    a. Diabetic coma
    b. Insulin coma
    c. Diabetic shock
    d. Insulin shock

69. The signs and symptoms of CHF include:

    a. increased appetite, profuse perspiration, frequent urination, and tremors in the extremities.
    b. weight loss, shallow respirations, dry skin, and constricted pupils.
    c. chest pain, tremors, redness of face and lips, and constricted pupils.
    d. severe fatigue, noisy respirations, profuse perspiration, and swelling of the ankles and feet.

70. What disorder of the cardiovascular system is caused by a sudden blockage of the coronary arteries?

    a. Angina pectoris
    b. Heart attack
    c. CHF
    d. CVA

71. Which of the following is another term for cerebrovascular accident?

    a. Hemorrhagic shock
    b. Angina pectoris
    c. Myocardial infarction
    d. Stroke

72. A common reaction in an amphetamine abuser who recently has had a "fix" is:

    a. drowsiness, lapsing into a light sleep.
    b. hallucinations, tremors, and convulsions.
    c. a trancelike state.
    d. nervousness, irritability, and increased activity.

73. A 40-year-old man experienced brief distress from chest pain to the left of his sternum. The pain occurred immediately after raking leaves in the yard. When you arrive, he no longer has any pain, but he is shaken by the episode. What disorder do these symptoms indicate?

    a. Heart attack
    b. Angina pectoris
    c. CHF
    d. Nervous exhaustion

74. A workman in a warm and humid boiler room is found in a state of collapse. He exhibits no signs of injury but has hot, dry skin. You should suspect he is suffering from heat:
    a. exhaustion.
    b. prostration.
    c. stroke.
    d. cramps.

75. A frostbitten extremity should be rewarmed by immersing it in a water bath within the temperature range of:
    a. 84 to 88 degrees F.
    b. 93 to 98 degrees F.
    c. 100 to 105 degrees F.
    d. 105 to 112 degrees F.

76. Anaphylactic shock is considered a true emergency in:
    a. very few persons.
    b. any person.
    c. a sensitized person only.
    d. cases of bee stings only.

77. A child has suffered third-degree burns on his abdomen, chest, and the front of both arms. The area that this burn covers is approximately:
    a. 10 percent.
    b. 20 percent.
    c. 27 percent.
    d. 30 percent.

78. Cherry red skin indicates:
    a. low blood pressure.
    b. anoxia.
    c. internal bleeding.
    d. carbon monoxide poisoning.

79. A chemical burn to the eye from a strong acid should be treated by:
    a. irrigating with a mild acid such as vinegar.
    b. irrigating with a mild base.
    c. irrigating from the bridge of the nose through the eye with water.
    d. covering both eyes with moist patches but do not irrigate.

80. The point of entry and exit for a patient suffering from electric shock should be treated with:
    a. Vaseline-impregnated dressings.
    b. moist dressings.
    c. dry dressings.
    d. left uncovered.

81. A third-degree burn should be treated by:
    a. covering it with a moist sterile dressing.
    b. covering it with a dry sterile dressing.
    c. pulling any remaining fabric from the burn site before bandaging.
    d. leaving uncovered to facilitate drying of the tissues.

82. A dry chemical burn from an unknown chemical should be treated by:
    a. washing it away with water.
    b. brushing the chemical away and then washing the site.
    c. brushing away the chemical and then bandaging the site.
    d. neutralizing with another chemical before washing or irrigating with water.

83. A woman who is pregnant for the first time is experiencing steady labor pains every 5 minutes. You should:
    a. prepare for immediate delivery and do not try to move the woman.
    b. transport the woman to a hospital for delivery there.
    c. hold the woman's legs together until arrival at the hospital.
    d. tell the woman to relax between contractions and to save her strength.

84. If there are no pulsations in an umbilical cord which delivers before the baby, the EMT should:
    a. gently push the umbilical cord back into the vagina.
    b. place a sterile gauze with a hole for the cord against the vaginal opening.
    c. gently push up on the baby's head through the cervix, but do not push the cord back into the vagina.
    d. wait for crowning to occur and deliver as a normal birth.

85. During a breech delivery where the head has not delivered within 3 minutes after the body, the EMT must:
    a. apply pressure over the mother's lower abdomen.
    b. gently pull the baby from the vagina.
    c. rush the baby and mother to the hospital.
    d. establish an airway for the baby.

86. If a baby is delivered still enclosed in the "bag of waters," the EMT should:
    a. rush the baby and mother to the hospital.
    b. cut the umbilical cord.

c. puncture the bag and remove the membrane from the area of the mouth and nose.
d. proceed with the delivery in a normal manner, since the bag will not present a problem.

87. In a normal delivery, the newborn's head is the presenting part. What is the usual crowning position of the head?
   a. Face down
   b. Face to the left
   c. Face to the right
   d. Face up

88. Abortion or miscarriage describes a delivery that occurs before how many weeks of the pregnancy?
   a. 20
   b. 28
   c. 32
   d. 26

89. After the delivery of the baby, the EMT should wait no longer than how many minutes for the delivery of the placenta?
   a. 30 seconds
   b. 1 minute
   c. 20 minutes
   d. 1 hour

90. A disadvantage of scoop-style stretchers is that:
   a. both sides of the patient must be accessible to apply the splint.
   b. they are too narrow.
   c. they are not adjustable for length.
   d. the patient may slip when carrying the device down a staircase.

91. How should an accident victim be pulled to safety?
   a. Along the side axis of the body
   b. Along the short axis of the body
   c. Along the long axis of the body
   d. On an angle away from the point of injury

92. In what position should an accident victim with a mild, closed head injury, but without signs of spinal injury, be placed to facilitate drainage and maintain an open airway?
   a. Supine, with the head tilted up
   b. Supine, with the extremities elevated and the face up
   c. Prone, with the head turned to the side
   d. Upper body elevated

93. In what position should an unconscious stroke victim be transported?
   a. On the back with the feet elevated
   b. On the side, with no pillow
   c. Seated, with the head tilted back and legs elevated
   d. Supine

94. In what position should you transport a sucking chest wound patient after the wound has been stabilized?
   a. Supine
   b. Prone
   c. Lying on the injured side
   d. Lying on the uninjured side

95. Care for mentally disturbed patients usually is provided under the laws of:
   a. actual consent.
   b. implied consent.
   c. informed consent.

96. If the parents or legal guardians of an injured minor child cannot be found within a reasonable time, and the child has sustained life-threatening injuries, the EMT may assume:
   a. actual consent is granted.
   b. consent is refused.
   c. implied consent is granted.
   d. informed consent is granted.

97. Before starting the secondary survey, the EMT should always:
   a. check the blood pressure.
   b. check the pulse and respiration rates.
   c. look the patient over for signs of deterioration.
   d. wait until all necessary equipment is ready.

98. An EMT normally measures the blood pressure by placing a blood pressure cuff over which artery?
   a. Carotid
   b. Brachial
   c. Femoral
   d. Radial

99. Which of the following conditions requires the most immediate attention?
   a. Open chest wound
   b. Multiple fractures
   c. Labor contractions 8 minutes apart
   d. First-degree burns of the back and legs

**100.** Upon arrival at the scene, the EMT should:
   a. run in without equipment to access the situation first.
   b. stay alert and begin to gather information.
   c. assist the driver in backing the ambulance as close to the door as possible before going on.
   d. do not rely on dispatch information to decide what equipment to bring in.

# ANSWERS

## CHAPTER 1

| QUESTION | ANSWER | PAGE REFERENCE | |
|---|---|---|---|
| | | *Emergency Care, 5th Ed.* | *Emergency Care & Transport., 4th Ed.* |
| 1 | B | 11 | NA |
| 2 | B | 16 | 7 |
| 3 | D | 17 | 14 |
| 4 | C | 16 | 7 |
| 5 | B | 16 | 15 |
| 6 | C | 19 | 16 |
| 7 | C | 17 | 15 |
| 8 | A | 20 | 19 |
| 9 | B | 20 | 17 |
| 10 | C | 22 | NA |
| 11 | A | 18 | 16 |
| 12 | A | 19 | 16 |
| 13 | C | 21 | NA |
| 14 | D | 19 | 16 |
| 15 | B | 17 | 16 |
| 16 | D | 20 | NA |
| 17 | C | 17 | 16 |
| 18 | B | 19 | 18 |

NA = No Answer         * = Conflicting Answer

# CHAPTER 2

|  |  | PAGE REFERENCE | |
|---|---|---|---|
| QUESTION | ANSWER | Emergency Care, 5th Ed. | Emergency Care & Transport., 4th Ed. |
| 1 | B | 33 | NA |
| 2 | D | 34 | NA |
| 3 | C | 33 | 23 |
| 4 | D | 33 | 23 |
| 5 | C | 33 | 23 |
| 6 | D | 37 | 27 |
| 7 | C | 33 | 27 |
| 8 | A | 34 | NA |
| 9 | D | 37 | 27 |
| 10 | B | 37 | NA |
| 11 | D | 39 | NA |
| 12 | A | 39 | NA |
| 13 | C | 37 | 27 |
| 14 | B | 34 | NA |
| 15 | C | 38 | 28 |
| 16 | D | 39 | 26 |
| 17 | C | 41 | 28 |
| 18 | A | 41 | 28 |
| 19 | C | 41 | 28 |
| 20 | B | 34 | NA |
| 21 | C | 38 | 28 |
| 22 | A | 36 | 24 |
| 23 | C | 46 | 24 |
| 24 | A | 42 | NA |
| 25 | C | 46 | 28 |
| 26 | A | 46 | 30 |
| 27 | B | 46 | NA |
| 28 | A | 46 | 24 |
| 29 | C | 33 | 27 |
| 30 | D | 39 | NA |

NA = No Answer        * = Conflicting Answer

# CHAPTER 3

**PAGE REFERENCE**

| QUESTION | ANSWER | Emergency Care, 5th Ed. | Emergency Care & Transport., 4th Ed. |
|---|---|---|---|
| 1 | D | 63 | 35 |
| 2 | D | 64 | NA |
| 3 | B | 66 | NA |
| 4 | B | 63 | NA |
| 5 | A | 70 | 45 |
| 6 | D | 73 | NA |
| 7 | B | 75 | 37 |
| 8 | C | 65 | 44 |
| 9 | A | 71 | 78 |
| 10 | D | 71 | * |
| 11 | B | 76 | * |
| 12 | B | 64 | NA |
| 13 | D | 71 | NA |
| 14 | A | 72 | 35 |
| 15 | C | 75 | NA |
| 16 | C | 65 | NA |
| 17 | B | 70 | 45 |
| 18 | C | 72 | 80 |
| 19 | B | 79 | 376 |
| 20 | D | 72 | NA |
| 21 | C | 73 | NA |
| 22 | A | 75 | NA |
| 23 | A | 63 | NA |
| 24 | C | 90 | NA |
| 25 | A | 82 | NA |
| 26 | A | 85 | 36 |
| 27 | D | 86 | NA |
| 28 | C | 80 | NA |
| 29 | D | 85 | NA |
| 30 | C | 88 | 38 |
| 31 | C | 86 | NA |
| 32 | A | 80 | 49 |
| 33 | C | 77 | NA |
| 34 | D | 85 | NA |
| 35 | B | 88 | 37 |
| 36 | A | 87 | 36 |
| 37 | D | 88 | NA |
| 38 | A | 94 | 41 |
| 39 | B | 95 | 53 |
| 40 | C | 88 | 38 |
| 41 | A | 88 | NA |
| 42 | B | 88 | NA |
| 43 | D | 88 | 38 |
| 44 | A | 88 | NA |
| 45 | B | 88 | 38 |
| 46 | C | 90 | 39 |
| 47 | D | 94 | 41 |
| 48 | A | 62 | NA |
| 49 | C | 91 | NA |
| 50 | B | 100 | NA |

NA = No Answer          * = Conflicting Answer

# CHAPTER 4

| QUESTION | ANSWER | PAGE REFERENCE *Emergency Care, 5th Ed.* | *Emergency Care & Transport., 4th Ed.* |
|---|---|---|---|
| 1 | B | 115 | 71 |
| 2 | C | 126 | 87 |
| 3 | B | 114 | 69 |
| 4 | B | 114 | 68 |
| 5 | C | 132 | 89 |
| 6 | A | 115 | 71 |
| 7 | C | 126 | NA |
| 8 | B | 121 | 77 |
| 9 | C | 122 | 82 |
| 10 | A | 112 | NA |
| 11 | C | 125 | NA |
| 12 | D | 126 | NA |
| 13 | A | 122 | 88 |
| 14 | B | 112 | 76 |
| 15 | A | 126 | 84 |
| 16 | A | 124 | 88 |
| 17 | C | 115 | 71 |
| 18 | C | 112 | 69 |
| 19 | D | 121 | NA |
| 20 | C | 126 | NA |
| 21 | C | 122 | 87 |
| 22 | C | 123 | 82 |
| 23 | B | 126 | NA |
| 24 | C | 114 | NA |
| 25 | B | 120 | 75 |
| 26 | A | 121 | 81 |
| 27 | B | 116 | NA |
| 28 | B | 116 | NA |
| 29 | A | 120 | NA |
| 30 | A | 112 | 69 |
| 31 | C | 112 | 70 |
| 32 | B | 115 | NA |
| 33 | B | 116 | NA |
| 34 | D | 116 | 77 |
| 35 | B | 114 | NA |
| 36 | D | 119 | 80 |
| 37 | A | 127 | 79 |
| 38 | A | 114 | 69 |
| 39 | B | 112 | 68 |
| 40 | A | 112 | 114 |
| 41 | D | 117 | 79 |

NA = No Answer         * = Conflicting Answer

# CHAPTER 5

|  |  | PAGE REFERENCE | |
|---|---|---|---|
| QUESTION | ANSWER | *Emergency Care, 5th Ed.* | *Emergency Care & Transport., 4th Ed.* |
| 1 | C | 138 | NA |
| 2 | C | 139 | NA |
| 3 | A | 143 | 100 |
| 4 | C | 141 | 75 |
| 5 | A | 141 | 101 |
| 6 | A | 145 | 102 |
| 7 | B | 141 | NA |
| 8 | C | 144 | 103 |
| 9 | A | 147 | 103 |
| 10 | B | 146 | 105 |
| 11 | C | 149 | NA |
| 12 | A | 148 | NA |
| 13 | D | 143 | 100 |
| 14 | A | 145 | 103 |
| 15 | D | 139 | 93 |
| 16 | B | 139 | 66 |
| 17 | C | 139 | NA |
| 18 | B | 140 | NA |
| 19 | A | 141 | NA |
| 20 | A | 145 | 103 |
| 21 | A | 145 | 103 |
| 22 | A | 146 | 105 |
| 23 | D | 141 | 100 |
| 24 | D | 138 | 99 |
| 25 | A | 144 | 102 |
| 26 | C | 155 | 106 |
| 27 | C | 147 | 102 |
| 28 | B | 138 | NA |
| 29 | C | 155 | NA |
| 30 | D | 155 | 106 |
| 31 | B | 156 | 107 |
| 32 | B | 144 | 102 |
| 33 | D | 141 | NA |
| 34 | B | 141 | 100 |
| 35 | C | 155 | 106 |
| 36 | C | 155 | 106 |
| 37 | B | 156 | 107 |
| 38 | D | 155 | * |
| 39 | C | 156 | NA |
| 40 | B | 156 | 107 |
| 41 | A | 155 | 107 |

*(continued)*

# CHAPTER 5 (Continued)

| QUESTION | ANSWER | PAGE REFERENCE *Emergency Care, 5th Ed.* | *Emergency Care & Transport., 4th Ed.* |
|---|---|---|---|
| 42 | C | 156 | 107 |
| 43 | C | 155 | 106 |
| 44 | D | 149 | 104 |
| 45 | C | 152 | 104 |
| 46 | B | 152 | 104 |
| 47 | C | 152 | NA |
| 48 | C | 152 | 104 |
| 49 | C | 146 | NA |
| 50 | A | 152 | * |
| 51 | B | 152 | 104 |
| 52 | A | 156 | 107 |
| 53 | B | 139 | NA |
| 54 | B | 140 | NA |
| 55 | C | 140 | NA |
| 56 | C | 139 | NA |
| 57 | C | 145 | 102 |
| 58 | A | 143 | NA |
| 59 | D | 143 | 80 |
| 60 | C | 147 | 103 |
| 61 | B | 147 | 102 |
| 62 | C | 149 | NA |
| 63 | B | 139 | NA |
| 64 | B | 143 | 100 |
| 65 | D | 146 | 105 |
| 66 | C | 148 | 105 |
| 67 | C | 146 | 105 |
| 68 | A | 143 | NA |
| 69 | B | 148 | NA |
| 70 | A | 143 | 100 |
| 71 | A | 156 | 107 |
| 72 | A | 152 | 104 |
| 73 | C | 147 | 103 |
| 74 | B | 147 | NA |
| 75 | D | 141 | NA |
| 76 | D | 139 | 92 |
| 77 | C | 142 | 100 |
| 78 | C | 147 | NA |
| 79 | B | 155 | 106 |
| 80 | A | 158 | NA |

NA = No Answer   * = Conflicting Answer

## CHAPTER 6

|  |  | PAGE REFERENCE | |
|---|---|---|---|
| QUESTION | ANSWER | *Emergency Care, 5th Ed.* | *Emergency Care & Transport., 4th Ed.* |
| 1 | C | 163 | 110 |
| 2 | B | 168 | 114 |
| 3 | C | 171 | NA |
| 4 | A | 162 | NA |
| 5 | C | 165 | 110 |
| 6 | D | 171 | NA |
| 7 | D | 162 | NA |
| 8 | B | 178 | 118 |
| 9 | C | 165 | 111 |
| 10 | C | 142 | * |
| 11 | A | 173 | 108 |
| 12 | B | 183 | NA |
| 13 | D | 166 | NA |
| 14 | B | 172 | 112 |
| 15 | C | 175 | 115 |
| 16 | A | 176 | 119 |
| 17 | D | 169 | NA |
| 18 | C | 170 | * |
| 19 | A | 175 | NA |
| 20 | C | 173 | NA |
| 21 | D | 174 | NA |
| 22 | B | 176 | NA |
| 23 | A | 178 | 117 |
| 24 | A | 164 | NA |
| 25 | C | 176 | 119 |
| 26 | B | 180 | NA |
| 27 | C | 181 | 120 |
| 28 | C | 171 | NA |
| 29 | D | 181 | 120 |
| 30 | A | 170 | NA |
| 31 | D | 183 | 122 |
| 32 | C | 163 | NA |
| 33 | D | 174 | 108 |
| 34 | C | 181 | * |
| 35 | B | 181 | NA |
| 36 | A | 174 | NA |
| 37 | A | 181 | NA |
| 38 | A | 177 | 117 |
| 39 | A | 181 | NA |
| 40 | B | 181 | * |

NA = No Answer        * = Conflicting Answer

## CHAPTER 7 — SECTION ONE

**PAGE REFERENCE**

| QUESTION | ANSWER | Emergency Care, 5th Ed. | Emergency Care & Transport., 4th Ed. |
|---|---|---|---|
| 1 | B | 193 | NA |
| 2 | A | 198 | NA |
| 3 | C | 206 | 135 |
| 4 | B | 203 | 135 |
| 5 | C | 206 | 138 |
| 6 | D | 203 | 136 |
| 7 | A | 194 | 124 |
| 8 | B | 199 | 127 |
| 9 | B | 201 | 131 |
| 10 | D | 203 | 136 |
| 11 | C | 195 | NA |
| 12 | B | 203 | 137 |
| 13 | C | 196 | NA |
| 14 | C | 193 | NA |
| 15 | B | 203 | 136 |
| 16 | B | 202 | NA |
| 17 | B | 203 | 135 |
| 18 | A | 205 | 138 |
| 19 | B | 208 | NA |
| 20 | C | 204 | 138 |
| 21 | D | 195 | NA |
| 22 | A | 194 | 134 |
| 23 | A | 203 | 137 |
| 24 | C | 201 | NA |
| 25 | D | 202 | 134 |
| 26 | D | 208 | 137 |
| 27 | A | 207 | 137 |
| 28 | D | 193 | NA |
| 29 | C | 198 | NA |
| 30 | A | 202 | 134 |
| 31 | C | 203 | 136 |
| 32 | A | 198 | 126 |
| 33 | C | 197 | 156 |
| 34 | A | 196 | 125 |
| 35 | B | 200 | 127 |
| 36 | D | 203 | 136 |
| 37 | A | 194 | 124 |
| 38 | D | 195 | 125 |
| 39 | A | 193 | NA |
| 40 | C | 204 | 138 |
| 41 | A | 203 | 136 |
| 42 | B | 203 | 137 |
| 43 | B | 192 | NA |

NA = No Answer          * = Conflicting Answer

## CHAPTER 7 — SECTION TWO

| QUESTION | ANSWER | PAGE REFERENCE *Emergency Care, 5th Ed.* | *Emergency Care & Transport., 4th Ed.* |
|---|---|---|---|
| 1 | C | 211 | 128 |
| 2 | D | 212 | * |
| 3 | B | 212 | 128 |
| 4 | A | 214 | 130 |
| 5 | D | 214 | 129 |
| 6 | B | 214 | * |
| 7 | D | 213 | 129 |
| 8 | A | 213 | * |

NA = No Answer     * = Conflicting Answer

## CHAPTER 8

| QUESTION | ANSWER | PAGE REFERENCE *Emergency Care, 5th Ed.* | *Emergency Care & Transport., 4th Ed.* |
|---|---|---|---|
| 1 | B | 219 | 151 |
| 2 | A | 222 | 153 |
| 3 | B | 218 | 154 |
| 4 | D | 218 | 160 |
| 5 | D | 227 | 155 |
| 6 | B | 232 | NA |
| 7 | A | 218 | NA |
| 8 | D | 221 | 154 |
| 9 | A | 223 | 154 |
| 10 | B | 224 | 159 |
| 11 | C | 219 | 151 |
| 12 | C | 226 | NA |
| 13 | C | 228 | 157 |
| 14 | D | 220 | 152 |
| 15 | D | 222 | 155 |
| 16 | D | 220 | NA |
| 17 | B | 222 | 154 |
| 18 | C | 225 | 161 |
| 19 | A | 228 | 159 |
| 20 | B | 228 | 158 |
| 21 | B | 221 | 152 |
| 22 | B | 226 | 156 |
| 23 | C | 230 | 157 |
| 24 | C | 220 | 152 |
| 25 | C | 224 | NA |
| 26 | C | 230 | NA |
| 27 | A | 228 | NA |
| 28 | C | 222 | 154 |
| 29 | A | 225 | 161 |
| 30 | A | 221 | 152 |

NA = No Answer     * = Conflicting Answer

## CHAPTER 9

| QUESTION | ANSWER | PAGE REFERENCE | |
|---|---|---|---|
| | | *Emergency Care, 5th Ed.* | *Emergency Care & Transport., 4th Ed.* |
| 1 | D | 237 | 187 |
| 2 | B | 243 | 171 |
| 3 | D | 239 | 164 |
| 4 | A | 247 | 184 |
| 5 | A | 247 | 183 |
| 6 | B | 247 | 184 |
| 7 | A | 250 | 184 |
| 8 | A | 239 | 180 |
| 9 | B | 245 | 187 |
| 10 | B | 256 | NA |
| 11 | B | 250 | 194 |
| 12 | B | 247 | 190 |
| 13 | A | 236 | 167 |
| 14 | A | 243 | 173 |
| 15 | C | 256 | 204 |
| 16 | C | 263 | 172 |
| 17 | B | 243 | 183 |
| 18 | A | 253 | 201 |
| 19 | A | 262 | 164 |
| 20 | C | 253 | 201 |
| 21 | C | 264 | 190 |
| 22 | C | 264 | 173 |
| 23 | B | 253 | NA |
| 24 | B | 257 | 196 |
| 25 | A | 260 | 168 |
| 26 | B | 239 | 184 |
| 27 | C | 248 | 179 |
| 28 | D | 263 | NA |
| 29 | B | 244 | 184 |
| 30 | B | 239 | NA |
| 31 | A | 263 | 185 |

NA = No Answer        * = Conflicting Answer

## CHAPTER 10

| QUESTION | ANSWER | PAGE REFERENCE | |
|---|---|---|---|
| | | *Emergency Care, 5th Ed.* | *Emergency Care & Transport., 4th Ed.* |
| 1 | C | 274 | 208 |
| 2 | C | 275 | 209 |
| 3 | A | 271 | 210 |
| 4 | D | 269 | 210 |
| 5 | B | 272 | 188 |
| 6 | D | 280 | 188 |
| 7 | B | 276 | 212 |
| 8 | B | 276 | 212 |

NA = No Answer        * = Conflicting Answer

# CHAPTER 11

**PAGE REFERENCE**

| QUESTION | ANSWER | Emergency Care, 5th Ed. | Emergency Care & Transport., 4th Ed. |
|---|---|---|---|
| 1 | B | 296 | NA |
| 2 | C | 297 | NA |
| 3 | D | 296 | 233 |
| 4 | B | 296 | NA |
| 5 | A | 299 | NA |
| 6 | A | 296 | NA |
| 7 | D | 297 | 232 |
| 8 | C | 299 | NA |
| 9 | B | 301 | 228 |
| 10 | B | 299 | 228 |
| 11 | C | 308 | 224 |
| 12 | A | 302 | 229 |
| 13 | A | 300 | 227 |
| 14 | B | 297 | 232 |
| 15 | B | 299 | NA |
| 16 | A | 300 | NA |
| 17 | C | 297 | 232 |
| 18 | A | 312 | 235 |
| 19 | A | 312 | NA |
| 20 | B | 309 | NA |
| 21 | B | 297 | 232 |
| 22 | B | 308 | NA |

NA = No Answer     * = Conflicting Answer

## CHAPTER 12

| QUESTION | ANSWER | PAGE REFERENCE | |
|---|---|---|---|
| | | *Emergency Care, 5th Ed.* | *Emergency Care & Transport., 4th Ed.* |
| 1 | C | 329 | 225 |
| 2 | A | 340 | NA |
| 3 | B | 343 | NA |
| 4 | B | 332 | 244 |
| 5 | C | 337 | 249 |
| 6 | A | 340 | 228 |
| 7 | A | 336 | 246 |
| 8 | A | 340 | 228 |
| 9 | C | 345 | 226 |
| 10 | B | 328 | 251 |
| 11 | C | 332 | 244 |
| 12 | A | 341 | 252 |
| 13 | A | 332 | 244 |
| 14 | C | 336 | 247 |
| 15 | A | 332 | 244 |
| 16 | C | 337 | 248 |
| 17 | B | 341 | 129 |
| 18 | A | 342 | NA |
| 19 | B | 341 | 129 |
| 20 | D | 338 | 250 |
| 21 | D | 341 | 252 |
| 22 | B | 332 | 244 |
| 23 | C | 343 | NA |
| 24 | D | 334 | 246 |
| 25 | A | 332 | 248 |
| 26 | B | 342 | 252 |
| 27 | B | 344 | 253 |
| 28 | C | 330 | 252 |
| 29 | A | 345 | 249 |
| 30 | C | 342 | 228 |
| 31 | B | 332 | 248 |
| 32 | A | 343 | 252 |
| 33 | D | 345 | NA |
| 34 | A | 344 | NA |
| 35 | B | 338 | 250 |
| 36 | C | 345 | NA |
| 37 | C | 333 | 248 |
| 38 | A | 328 | 225 |
| 39 | B | 332 | 253 |
| 40 | C | 328 | 252 |
| 41 | B | 332 | 252 |

NA = No Answer       * = Conflicting Answer

## CHAPTER 13

|  |  | PAGE REFERENCE | |
|---|---|---|---|
| QUESTION | ANSWER | *Emergency Care, 5th Ed.* | *Emergency Care & Transport., 4th Ed.* |
| 1 | C | 360 | 266 |
| 2 | A | 360 | 266 |
| 3 | A | 363 | 277 |
| 4 | A | 363 | 279 |
| 5 | C | 360 | 266 |
| 6 | B | 362 | 279 |
| 7 | A | 362 | 279 |
| 8 | A | 366 | 279 |
| 9 | B | 361 | 278 |
| 10 | D | 350 | 260 |
| 11 | B | 350 | 258 |
| 12 | C | 359 | 261 |
| 13 | C | 359 | 263 |
| 14 | D | 357 | 258 |
| 15 | C | 354 | 261 |
| 16 | D | 359 | NA |
| 17 | B | 354 | NA |
| 18 | C | 355 | 256 |
| 19 | B | 355 | 257 |
| 20 | A | 355 | 257 |
| 21 | A | 356 | 257 |

NA = No Answer         * = Conflicting Answer

# CHAPTER 14 — SECTION ONE

**PAGE REFERENCE**

| QUESTION | ANSWER | *Emergency Care, 5th Ed.* | *Emergency Care & Transport., 4th Ed.* |
|---|---|---|---|
| 1 | A | 397 | * |
| 2 | B | 387 | 309 |
| 3 | C | 388 | 310 |
| 4 | C | 373 | NA |
| 5 | D | 392 | 313 |
| 6 | D | 388 | 310 |
| 7 | C | 372 | 327 |
| 8 | D | 387 | 343 |
| 9 | C | 388 | 313 |
| 10 | D | 372 | NA |
| 11 | C | 392 | 316 |
| 12 | C | 394 | NA |
| 13 | C | 394 | 329 |
| 14 | A | 399 | 325 |
| 15 | B | 394 | 319 |
| 16 | C | 387 | 317 |
| 17 | B | 393 | 313 |
| 18 | D | 392 | 312 |
| 19 | A | 392 | 322 |
| 20 | A | 394 | 334 |
| 21 | C | 399 | NA |
| 22 | A | 372 | 320 |
| 23 | C | 387 | 309 |
| 24 | A | 386 | 319 |
| 25 | D | 394 | 328 |
| 26 | C | 398 | 311 |
| 27 | B | 388 | 287 |
| 28 | D | 371 | 312 |
| 29 | B | 392 | 319 |
| 30 | C | 394 | 312 |
| 31 | C | 392 | NA |
| 32 | A | 396 | 316 |
| 33 | A | 393 | 317 |
| 34 | D | 394 | 327 |
| 35 | C | 398 | 322 |
| 36 | C | 395 | NA |
| 37 | D | 375 | 298 |
| 38 | B | 380 | NA |
| 39 | A | 381 | 301 |
| 40 | D | 375 | 291 |
| 41 | D | 381 | 292 |
| 42 | C | 374 | 293 |
| 43 | C | 376 | 293 |
| 44 | A | NA | 292 |
| 45 | C | 377 | 293 |
| 46 | A | 377 | 293 |
| 47 | B | 413 | 369 |
| 48 | B | NA | * |
| 49 | C | 379 | 293 |

NA = No Answer    * = Conflicting Answer

## CHAPTER 14 — SECTION TWO

| | | PAGE REFERENCE | |
|---|---|---|---|
| QUESTION | ANSWER | *Emergency Care, 5th Ed.* | *Emergency Care & Transport., 4th Ed.* |
| 1 | B | 404 | 337 |
| 2 | C | 403 | 336 |
| 3 | C | 404 | 337 |
| 4 | A | 408 | 340 |
| 5 | C | 404 | 337 |
| 6 | B | 370 | NA |
| 7 | B | 403 | 335 |
| 8 | B | 403 | 336 |
| 9 | A | 406 | 381 |
| 10 | A | 411 | 366 |
| 11 | B | 412 | 368 |
| 12 | D | 412 | 367 |
| 13 | B | 412 | NA |
| 14 | C | 414 | 371 |

NA = No Answer          * = Conflicting Answer

## CHAPTER 15

| | | PAGE REFERENCE | |
|---|---|---|---|
| QUESTION | ANSWER | *Emergency Care, 5th Ed.* | *Emergency Care & Transport., 4th Ed.* |
| 1 | D | 422 | 394 |
| 2 | C | 422 | NA |
| 3 | B | 420 | NA |
| 4 | C | 430 | 390 |
| 5 | A | 418 | 384 |
| 6 | B | 420 | NA |
| 7 | C | 421 | NA |
| 8 | B | 428 | NA |
| 9 | B | 428 | NA |
| 10 | B | 422 | NA |
| 11 | D | 421 | NA |
| 12 | C | 424 | 391 |
| 13 | B | 431 | NA |
| 14 | B | 421 | 392 |
| 15 | D | 426 | 384 |
| 16 | D | 427 | NA |
| 17 | D | 422 | 385 |
| 18 | B | 428 | * |
| 19 | A | 421 | 385 |
| 20 | B | 428 | 389 |

NA = No Answer          * = Conflicting Answer

# CHAPTER 16

|  |  | PAGE REFERENCE | |
|---|---|---|---|
| QUESTION | ANSWER | *Emergency Care, 5th Ed.* | *Emergency Care & Transport., 4th Ed.* |
| 1 | B | 436 | 396 |
| 2 | B | 439 | * |
| 3 | D | 442 | 405 |
| 4 | B | 450 | 404 |
| 5 | A | 437 | 396 |
| 6 | B | 440 | 398 |
| 7 | D | 446 | NA |
| 8 | A | 450 | 408 |
| 9 | C | 436 | 397 |
| 10 | C | 442 | 402 |
| 11 | A | 447 | 404 |
| 12 | B | 450 | NA |
| 13 | D | 436 | 397 |
| 14 | D | 440 | * |
| 15 | C | 451 | 396 |
| 16 | A | 436 | 396 |
| 17 | B | 442 | 402 |
| 18 | B | 446 | * |
| 19 | C | 452 | 353 |
| 20 | B | 447 | 404 |
| 21 | C | 445 | 405 |
| 22 | D | 452 | * |
| 23 | C | 436 | 396 |
| 24 | B | 445 | 405 |
| 25 | B | 436 | NA |
| 26 | B | 453 | NA |
| 27 | C | 454 | 407 |
| 28 | D | 436 | 398 |
| 29 | A | 444 | * |
| 30 | C | 448 | NA |
| 31 | D | 454 | 407 |
| 32 | A | 436 | NA |
| 33 | C | 442 | 400 |
| 34 | D | 449 | NA |
| 35 | A | 455 | * |
| 36 | C | 453 | 406 |
| 37 | B | 442 | 400 |
| 38 | A | 449 | 405 |
| 39 | C | 456 | 410 |
| 40 | C | 438 | 404 |
| 41 | D | 442 | 401 |
| 42 | A | 439 | NA |
| 43 | D | 447 | 405 |
| 44 | D | 449 | 406 |

NA = No Answer        * = Conflicting Answer

## CHAPTER 17

| QUESTION | ANSWER | PAGE REFERENCE | |
|---|---|---|---|
| | | *Emergency Care, 5th Ed.* | *Emergency Care & Transport., 4th Ed.* |
| 1 | A | 461 | 413 |
| 2 | B | 463 | 414 |
| 3 | B | 461 | 414 |
| 4 | C | 461 | 418 |
| 5 | D | 470 | 418 |
| 6 | D | 471 | 427 |
| 7 | A | 461 | 413 |
| 8 | D | 461 | 414 |
| 9 | D | 463 | 415 |
| 10 | B | 474 | 422 |
| 11 | C | 465 | 415 |
| 12 | A | 468 | 417 |
| 13 | C | 463 | 415 |
| 14 | A | 477 | NA |
| 15 | C | 468 | 418 |
| 16 | B | 468 | 417 |
| 17 | B | 463 | 414 |
| 18 | B | 470 | 419 |

NA = No Answer        * = Conflicting Answer

## CHAPTER 18 — SECTION ONE

| QUESTION | ANSWER | PAGE REFERENCE | |
|---|---|---|---|
| | | *Emergency Care, 5th Ed.* | *Emergency Care & Transport., 4th Ed.* |
| 1 | B | 485 | NA |
| 2 | A | 482 | 431 |
| 3 | B | 488 | 435 |
| 4 | B | 481 | 431 |
| 5 | C | 487 | 434 |
| 6 | C | 488 | 434 |
| 7 | B | 481 | 432 |
| 8 | C | 486 | * |

NA = No Answer        * = Conflicting Answer

## CHAPTER 18 — SECTION TWO

### PAGE REFERENCE

| QUESTION | ANSWER | Emergency Care, 5th Ed. | Emergency Care & Transport., 4th Ed. |
|---|---|---|---|
| 1 | C | 494 | 439 |
| 2 | A | 491 | 439 |
| 3 | C | 496 | 442 |
| 4 | B | 494 | 438 |
| 5 | D | 498 | 439 |

NA = No Answer        * = Conflicting Answer

## CHAPTER 19

### PAGE REFERENCE

| QUESTION | ANSWER | Emergency Care, 5th Ed. | Emergency Care & Transport., 4th Ed. |
|---|---|---|---|
| 1 | B | 502 | 446 |
| 2 | A | 505 | 447 |
| 3 | D | 511 | 450 |
| 4 | A | 503 | NA |
| 5 | D | 506 | 447 |
| 6 | B | 511 | 451 |
| 7 | B | 506 | 448 |
| 8 | D | 511 | NA |
| 9 | A | 515 | NA |
| 10 | D | 502 | NA |
| 11 | B | 512 | 450 |
| 12 | C | 505 | 447 |
| 13 | A | 510 | NA |
| 14 | B | 513 | NA |
| 15 | C | 511 | 451 |

NA = No Answer        * = Conflicting Answer

## CHAPTER 20

| QUESTION | ANSWER | PAGE REFERENCE *Emergency Care, 5th Ed.* | *Emergency Care & Transport., 4th Ed.* |
|---|---|---|---|
| 1 | B | 518 | NA |
| 2 | C | 518 | 483 |
| 3 | B | 518 | 483 |
| 4 | A | 519 | NA |
| 5 | D | 519 | 483 |
| 6 | D | 518 | 481 |
| 7 | B | 518 | 483 |
| 8 | A | 518 | 483 |
| 9 | A | 518 | 483 |
| 10 | B | 518 | 483 |
| 11 | D | 519 | NA |
| 12 | B | 518 | 483 |
| 13 | A | 518 | 483 |
| 14 | D | 519 | 483 |
| 15 | D | 519 | NA |
| 16 | A | 518 | 483 |
| 17 | A | 518 | 483 |
| 18 | B | 518 | 483 |
| 19 | D | 526 | NA |
| 20 | A | 518 | 483 |

NA = No Answer       * = Conflicting Answer

## CHAPTER 21

| QUESTION | ANSWER | PAGE REFERENCE *Emergency Care, 5th Ed.* | *Emergency Care & Transport., 4th Ed.* |
|---|---|---|---|

None

## CHAPTER 22

**PAGE REFERENCE**

| QUESTION | ANSWER | Emergency Care, 5th Ed. | Emergency Care & Transport., 4th Ed. |
|---|---|---|---|
| 1 | D | 545 | NA |
| 2 | C | 551 | NA |
| 3 | A | 550 | NA |
| 4 | D | 559 | NA |
| 5 | B | 545 | 528 |
| 6 | B | 551 | NA |
| 7 | A | 546 | 531 |
| 8 | D | 559 | NA |
| 9 | A | 545 | NA |
| 10 | D | 547 | NA |
| 11 | A | 559 | 535 |
| 12 | D | 559 | NA |
| 13 | B | 546 | NA |
| 14 | C | 547 | NA |
| 15 | A | 562 | NA |
| 16 | A | 546 | NA |
| 17 | B | 546 | 531 |
| 18 | D | 559 | NA |

NA = No Answer        * = Conflicting Answer

## CHAPTER 23

**PAGE REFERENCE**

| QUESTION | ANSWER | Emergency Care, 5th Ed. | Emergency Care & Transport., 4th Ed. |
|---|---|---|---|
| 1 | A | 573 | NA |
| 2 | D | 579 | NA |
| 3 | D | 572 | NA |
| 4 | A | 581 | NA |
| 5 | B | 584 | 467 |
| 6 | D | 580 | 482 |
| 7 | B | 581 | NA |
| 8 | D | 581 | 476 |
| 9 | B | 580 | NA |
| 10 | B | 575 | 478 |
| 11 | C | 575 | 477 |
| 12 | A | 573 | NA |
| 13 | B | 575 | NA |
| 14 | B | 573 | NA |

NA = No Answer        * = Conflicting Answer

## CHAPTER 24

| QUESTION | ANSWER | PAGE REFERENCE | |
|---|---|---|---|
| | | *Emergency Care, 5th Ed.* | *Emergency Care & Transport., 4th Ed.* |
| 1 | B | 588 | NA |
| 2 | D | 589 | NA |
| 3 | A | 588 | NA |
| 4 | B | 589 | NA |
| 5 | D | 590 | NA |
| 6 | A | 588 | NA |
| 7 | C | 589 | NA |
| 8 | B | 588 | NA |
| 9 | C | 588 | NA |

NA = No Answer          * = Conflicting Answer

## CHAPTER 25

| QUESTION | ANSWER | PAGE REFERENCE | |
|---|---|---|---|
| | | *Emergency Care, 5th Ed.* | *Emergency Care & Transport., 4th Ed.* |

None

## CHAPTER 26

| QUESTION | ANSWER | PAGE REFERENCE | |
|---|---|---|---|
| | | *Emergency Care, 5th Ed.* | *Emergency Care & Transport., 4th Ed.* |
| 1 | C | 607 | 543 |
| 2 | B | 607 | 543 |
| 3 | C | 607 | NA |
| 4 | B | 607 | 543 |
| 5 | A | 609 | 548 |

NA = No Answer          * = Conflicting Answer

## CHAPTER 27 — SECTION ONE

| QUESTION | ANSWER | PAGE REFERENCE | |
|---|---|---|---|
| | | *Emergency Care, 5th Ed.* | *Emergency Care & Transport., 4th Ed.* |

None

## CHAPTER 27 — SECTION TWO

| QUESTION | ANSWER | PAGE REFERENCE *Emergency Care, 5th Ed.* | *Emergency Care & Transport., 4th Ed.* |
|---|---|---|---|
| 1 | C | 630 | NA |
| 2 | A | 630 | NA |
| 3 | C | 631 | NA |
| 4 | B | 639 | NA |
| 5 | B | 637 | 496 |

NA = No Answer     * = Conflicting Answer

## CHAPTER 27 — SECTION THREE

| QUESTION | ANSWER | PAGE REFERENCE *Emergency Care, 5th Ed.* | *Emergency Care & Transport., 4th Ed.* |
|---|---|---|---|
| 1 | D | 647 | 498 |
| 2 | A | 642 | NA |
| 3 | A | 645 | 498 |
| 4 | C | 645 | NA |

NA = No Answer     * = Conflicting Answer

## CHAPTER 27 — SECTION FOUR

| QUESTION | ANSWER | PAGE REFERENCE *Emergency Care, 5th Ed.* | *Emergency Care & Transport., 4th Ed.* |
|---|---|---|---|
| 1 | A | 653 | NA |
| 2 | B | 661 | 502 |
| 3 | D | 662 | NA |
| 4 | C | 663 | 501 |
| 5 | D | 656 | 501 |
| 6 | A | 653 | NA |
| 7 | B | 655 | NA |
| 8 | B | 658 | 501 |
| 9 | C | 662 | 502 |

NA = No Answer     * = Conflicting Answer

## CHAPTER 28 — FINAL EXAM

| QUESTION | ANSWER | PAGE REFERENCE *Emergency Care, 5th Ed.* | *Emergency Care & Transport., 4th Ed.* |
|---|---|---|---|
| 1 | B | 112 | 68 |
| 2 | A | 49 | 94 |
| 3 | A | 360 | 269 |
| 4 | D | 37 | 169 |
| 5 | C | 38 | 268 |
| 6 | D | 193 | 124 |
| 7 | C | 188 | 115 |
| 8 | C | 177 | 119 |
| 9 | B | 83 | 39 |
| 10 | A | 121 | NA |
| 11 | C | 398 | 332 |
| 12 | D | 121 | 80 |
| 13 | A | 126 | NA |
| 14 | D | 124 | 83 |
| 15 | C | 122 | 88 |
| 16 | A | 164 | NA |
| 17 | A | 155 | 106 |
| 18 | C | 145 | 103 |
| 19 | A | 145 | 103 |
| 20 | D | 143 | 100 |
| 21 | C | 143 | NA |
| 22 | C | 143 | 101 |
| 23 | B | 144 | 102 |
| 24 | B | 152 | 104 |
| 25 | C | 146 | 105 |
| 26 | D | 149 | NA |
| 27 | C | 206 | 138 |
| 28 | A | 203 | 135 |
| 29 | D | 207 | 139 |
| 30 | C | 203 | 136 |
| 31 | D | 200 | 127 |
| 32 | D | 208 | 137 |
| 33 | D | 224 | 140 |
| 34 | D | 345 | NA |
| 35 | B | 198 | 126 |
| 36 | C | 204 | 138 |
| 37 | C | 222 | 154 |
| 38 | C | 226 | NA |
| 39 | B | 345 | 158 |
| 40 | D | 230 | 157 |
| 41 | A | 354 | NA |
| 42 | B | 357 | 258 |
| 43 | B | 334 | 249 |
| 44 | C | 365 | 273 |
| 45 | A | 363 | NA |
| 46 | D | 362 | 157 |
| 47 | B | 276 | 210 |
| 48 | D | 265 | 201 |
| 49 | D | 264 | 190 |
| 50 | C | 253 | NA |
| 51 | B | 256 | 190 |

*(continued)*

# CHAPTER 28 — (Continued)

| QUESTION | ANSWER | PAGE REFERENCE | |
|---|---|---|---|
| | | Emergency Care, 5th Ed. | Emergency Care & Transport., 4th Ed. |
| 52 | A | 272 | NA |
| 53 | B | 247 | 183 |
| 54 | A | 340 | 229 |
| 55 | C | 302 | 41 |
| 56 | A | 306 | NA |
| 57 | C | 300 | 228 |
| 58 | A | 303 | 229 |
| 59 | D | 302 | 230 |
| 60 | B | 302 | * |
| 61 | D | 312 | 239 |
| 62 | D | 582 | NA |
| 63 | D | 579 | NA |
| 64 | A | 309 | 273 |
| 65 | C | 322 | 236 |
| 66 | C | 406 | 382 |
| 67 | C | 376 | 291 |
| 68 | A | 405 | 338 |
| 69 | D | 393 | 316 |
| 70 | B | 388 | 311 |
| 71 | D | 394 | 319 |
| 72 | D | 414 | 368 |
| 73 | B | 388 | 311 |
| 74 | C | 482 | 432 |
| 75 | C | 486 | 436 |
| 76 | B | 207 | NA |
| 77 | C | 463 | * |
| 78 | D | 378 | 417 |
| 79 | C | 336 | 418 |
| 80 | C | 470 | NA |
| 81 | A | 467 | * |
| 82 | B | 468 | 417 |
| 83 | B | 440 | NA |
| 84 | C | 454 | 408 |
| 85 | D | 453 | 407 |
| 86 | C | 442 | 405 |
| 87 | A | 442 | * |
| 88 | B | 452 | * |
| 89 | C | 447 | * |
| 90 | A | 573 | 480 |
| 91 | C | 584 | NA |
| 92 | D | 304 | 252 |
| 93 | B | 395 | 322 |
| 94 | C | 354 | NA |
| 95 | B | 20 | 16 |
| 96 | C | 19 | 16 |
| 97 | C | 97 | NA |
| 98 | B | 84 | 38 |
| 99 | A | 518 | 483 |
| 100 | B | 64 | NA |

NA = No Answer          * = Conflicting Answer